MW00744214

# Saving Our Sons
# & Daughters II

# Saving Our Sons & Daughters II

## Stories to uplift and educate the world about Duchenne Muscular Dystrophy

Misty VanderWeele presents
Saving Our Sons & Daughters II
along with 39 other Duchenne Authors and Contributors.

Publisher, Misty VanderWeele (MV International)
PO Box 4124
Palmer, Alaska 99645

Cover design by Killer Covers
Cover photography: Lori and Sam Safford by Kathy Mangum Photography www.kmangumphotography.com. The girl in the fountain, Carlie Frangela by mother Kelly Frangela.

Specially Autographed
For:

_The Aumine Family_

By:

_allan Love._

_Alice_ x _Nick_

_Pg 79_

# Acknowledgments

To each one of you, with all of my heart, I thank you:

- Glen, my husband and my "All of the Above", without your love and quiet, but strong support, I couldn't do what I do in the way that I do it.

- Jenna, my lovely and sensitive daughter, for your sincere understanding and love. As you grow up, I am in awe, and yes, "I Wish"!

- Luke, my son, for your friendship, love, and trust. You are the driving force behind my Duchenne Advocacy Mission. Seeing you thrive is incredible!

- Dr. Rhodes for creating a tool to aid in my son's healing, the STS/VECTTOR. Seeing Luke doing so well is a dream come true. Without Luke doing well, I couldn't devote as much time and energy to the Duchenne Movement. Your work will continue to change the Duchennne story, "our" story.

- All DMD daughters whose stories are included in this book, thank you for representing the very rare occurrence of Duchenne in girls and for teaching us so much. Your courage, bravery, and resolve to live life to the fullest despite having a rare disease, inspire us all.

- Lori Safford for all your hard work enriching this book project with your editing expertise, wisdom, friendship, and personal experience raising two handsome sons with DMD, while still managing to be there for your daughter. You don't miss a beat!

- My anonymous editor, as always, your generosity of time and support of my mission is heart touching.

- Star Babatoon for adding your professional yet positive loving energy to this book project.

- To CureDuchenne, Parent Project Muscular Dystrophy, FightDMD and all the other Duchenne organizations for your dedication to the Duchenne movement and believing in "our" story.

- To all my Facebook family and friends for your continued faith in me and stepping up your commitment to advocate for Duchenne until the whole world hears.

- To each and every co-author who shared their story. I am proud of your courage, love, and dedication in taking a stand for yourself, your children, and your loved ones.

- Angel in the fountain that graces the cover of this book. What a gift! I feel your wings of guardianship and protection. Your appearance strengths my resolve in taking our Duchenne story GLOBAL.

Saving Our Sons & Daughters II is dedicated to
all the Duchenne children, past, present and future;

*"While music is a universal language,
catastrophic illness and our stories
connect us to each other and to the World."*

*~Patricia Furlong,
Founder and CEO of
Parent Project Muscular Dystrophy*

# *Foreword*

Within the pages of *Saving Our Sons and Daughters II* are real life stories from parents, grandparents, siblings, and individuals living in the face of the most common, but unheard of, muscular dystrophy: Duchenne (DMD). DMD progressively robs the body of muscle, of air, of cardiac function, and eventually, of life. As I'm sure you know, without muscle our bodies would be just weak bags of bones, without the ability to stand. Our lungs would be squished flat with no way to expand and breath. Living would be impossible. Our sons, and some daughters, born seemingly healthy with almost no visible signs of the disease, begin the downward spiral of muscle wasting. Signs of Duchenne become apparent around 2 years of age and can go undiagnosed in some cases until the age of 8. Eventually, somewhere around 12 years of age, the use of a wheelchair becomes necessary. This transition into a wheelchair necessitates the purchase of an accessible van, home modifications and Individual Education Plans (IEPs) in school.

As the child reaches puberty, the muscles continue to deteriorate, contract, and weaken, the spine starts to curve causing scoliosis, in turn compromising the respiratory and immune systems. Cardiac function is next. All of these medical issues create the need for leg and back braces, leg and foot tendon release and spinal fusion surgeries, breathing equipment and sometimes, frequent hospital stays. Tragically, many of our children do not survive young adult hood.

There is nothing like the words *"there is no cure"* to strike fear within the hearts of parents, families and individuals themselves. This kind of fear is exactly what grips you when you are told your child has Duchenne Muscular Dystrophy. Not only does DMD have no cure, but parents are often times told to just take their children home and love them, because nothing can be done. Regardless if you have no idea what Duchenne is, or you know and love someone who is facing this horrid disease, you are in the right place at the right time. Duchenne families and individuals worldwide need your help right now. They need for you to understand what DMD is, how it is devastating their family, and then to go out and do something about it. Whether you can offer a shoulder to lean on, organize a major fundraising campaign, or simply learn to open doors for families and not to park in the handicap spots, you can do something to help. The point is, Duchenne needs global recognition. Though we are closer than ever before to effective treatments, we still need a cure. Each one of the families represented in this book is hoping for a cure in their child's lifetime. Education is sorely needed so that the world can wake up to this devastating disease. Sadly, children as young as 13 are dying from Duchenne. Something must be done to save our sons and daughters.

Duchenne affects approximately 1 in every 3500 live male births and it is caused by a missing protein called dystrophin. The disease is diagnosed by a genetic blood test which looks at the dystrophin gene. Females can have Duchenne as well, but it is considered rare. Not enough is yet known about the statistics of females affected. Some would even argue that girls can't have DMD, but blood tests prove otherwise. Out of the 38 family stories in this book, only two of them are about females. Because females are affected by DMD, the second part of this book's title is *and Daughters II*. In addition, females (moms and daughters) can be carriers of DMD. Women who are carriers have a 50% chance of having an affected child, but it is 50% for each child and in some cases, like the Saffords, that adds up to 100% of the Safford children. Although Duchenne can be inherited, about 35% of women are spontaneous carriers. There is also a small percentage of moms who are not carriers of Duchenne, but they have a child who has the disease. Duchenne can happen to any family.

As you turn the pages of this book, you will see that each story reveals a depth of love, courage, hope, and grace that only comes from living the nightmare that is Duchenne. Each parent watches DMD ravage their little child's body, powerless to stop the devastating effects. They live with the knowledge of what's to come, while doing everything in their power to give their child the best life they can. Most likely you will need a tissue or two, although I think many of the stories will surprise you. These families tell the horror story of Duchenne with humor, grace, and a positive outlook on life. These stories honor our sons and our daughters, because they are the true heroes in our lives.

The book unfolds based on the progression of muscle loss in Duchenne. The first section starts at six months and ends at age nine; the second section starts at age ten and ends at fifteen; the third at age fifteen and beyond. The book ends with five Duchenne stories and one poem from young adults who have not let Duchenne stop them from living.

Shortly after submitting her story, co-author Melaine Mackie's son, Dylan Smith, lost his battle with Duchenne at the tender age of 14. Please note the special page that we have dedicated to him.

We come before you now as advocates and parents who are no longer willing to swallow the *nothing can be done* pill. This mind set stops here! Together WE can make a difference!

# *Preface*

Whether we planned our children or they were planned for us, the love we have for these special gifts of life is indescribable. We never know how much we can love until we let a child into our hearts. After the first smile, we are forever hooked and would do almost anything to bring them joy and happiness. Alternatively, when that child suffers, there is no bottom to the depth of pain we feel.

Kahlil Gibran says "The deeper that sorrow carves into your being, the more joy you can contain." When you love a child with any life-altering disease, your sorrow runs deep. Deeper than you can ever imagine, but by the same token you have a deeper capacity for joy.

The focus of this book is not sorrow but joy. The purpose is to uplift the spirit and educate the world about Duchenne Muscular Dystrophy.

We all face challenges in life. As parents of children with DMD, we are not saying that our challenges are greater that anyone else's. What we are saying, with absolute certainty, is that we are greater than our challenges. As you read the following pages, you will see that we are strong, caring, sensitive and above all, human. What you will find is love, advocacy, and hope.

We hope that you will be touched by these stories and come away with a greater understanding of the human spirit, but we want more. We want you to be inspired and motivated to take action. Find a way to make a difference. Use any of the myriad of avenues created and sustained by the individual contributors of this book or find your own way to make a difference and spread awareness of DMD.

Cultural anthropologist Margaret Mead said "Never believe that a few caring people can't change the world. For, indeed, that's all who ever have." Be that caring person, do what you can to change the world of DMD and you will change the world at large.

Star Bobatoon
Attorney, Trainer, Author, Mother

Special Dedication to Dylan Smith who lost his battle to Duchenne during the creation of Saving Our Sons and Daughters II.

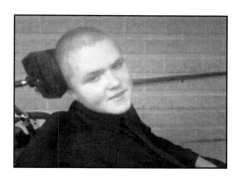

### *Heaven's Butterfly*

As I gaze out of the window,
My mind is full of missing you,
A tiny white butterfly dances,
Darting in and out of view,
A smile it starts to creep,
To my lips, my tears they cease,
This butterfly is dancing,
To remind me, to appease,
My love for you it's endless,
I don't have to let it go,
This twirling butterfly reminds me,
Love is eternal, warmth, a glow,
Missing you is inevitable,
It fills my waking hours, my day,
But loving you brings understanding,
Sadly that it has to be this way,
The butterfly from heaven shows me,
My Angel is thinking of me too,
So I'll smile at the beautiful butterfly,
Knowing my love flies up to you.,

~Unknown

*"You never know how strong you are until being strong is the only choice you have"*

*~Unknown*

# Contents

# Daniel, 6 Months Old

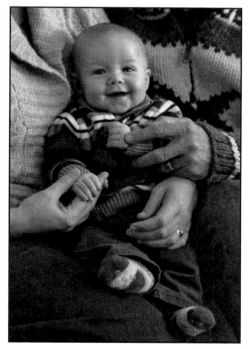

"Fearfully and wonderfully made" keeps ringing in my ears as I watch my sweet son sleep. Ten tiny fingers and toes, a perfect button sized nose. He gently touches me with his soft hands as he sleeps in my arms. I wonder what he dreams about as I see him smile, and almost giggle, in his sleep. Daniel was born in June of 2011. His birth mother had made the decision to give this precious child life but chose to have another family raise him. He was born in the middle of a hot June day via C-section.

All the regular tests were performed when the birth mother informed the staff that she had given birth to a son seven years ago with DMD. Immediately the medical staff ran a few tests and notified the chosen family of the health concerns. It must have been an incredible shock; they informed the hospital staff they would consider picking the baby up the next day. However, after what must have been a very long night of heart wrenching evaluation, they called the hospital to announce they would not be picking Daniel up from the hospital and did not feel they were the parents for him. The medical diagnosis of Duchenne Muscular Dystrophy (DMD) was just too much for them to bear.

The birth mother was given the names of several agencies and the option of picking another family. She decided to have her new agency choose the birth family. It was a Saturday morning when my husband and I were talking with our children about updating our adoption home study. After a year of hearing nothing we thought perhaps it wasn't the Lord's will to bless us with another child. We felt richly blessed with the ten children the Lord had given us; six born from us physically and four that had been born from our hearts through adoption. Our oldest son was soon to be wed and the thought occurred to us that perhaps, the season of having more children had come to a close.

Fifteen minutes after our family meeting we received an email from our attorney letting us know about Daniel and his need for a family. We instantly felt connected to this little boy. I still remember the adoption worker calling me to discuss Daniel's medical condition. She explained what DMD was and his expected life span, and then she said, "Well have I scarred you away yet?" I giggled and replied, "No, Not at all!" She continued to ask me more questions, took our home study, and then told me she would have an answer for me on who they chose to be the family for this sweet boy within the next few days. Those days were difficult for the entire family. I wanted more than anything to just know, "Is he my son?" It was with great joy that we answered the phone a few days later and received the answer; we would be Daniel's family.

By the end of the week we were at the agency picking up our son from the temporary home where he had been staying. The moment I saw him I could feel the tears welling up inside me; they were happy tears! God had given us the gift of another son! My husband and I were ushered into a private room where we sat admiring every detail of his tiny frame. Paperwork was signed, issues discussed, and appointments were made for the upcoming days. Joe and I left the agency and then spent several hours talking, praying, and thanking the Lord for this precious gift. Daniel was welcomed home by all 10 of his siblings. Each child enjoyed something special with Daniel. One child was the first to hold him, another was the one that picked out his "coming home" outfit, another child picked out his baby bedding, and so forth. Every member of the family was delighted that Daniel was home.

We quickly made an appointment with our family pediatrician. It was an excellent visit. We discussed expectations, asked questions, answered questions, and together we created a plan of care we believed to be in Daniel's best interest. Since Daniel had been discharged from the hospital a week prior, he had lost over a pound. We adjusted his bottle nipples, kept him slightly elevated while feeding, and then loved on him constantly. We took him back into the doctor a week after making these adjustments and were very happy with the results; Daniel had put on 16 of the 20 ounces he had previously lost. I'll never forget the nurse coming into the room after weighing Daniel. "Daniel's mom, I do believe it was love that put that pound of weight back on him!"

Daniel has continued to grow, slower than others, but steadily he grows. He is six months of age and has just started turning over. As my husband says, he may be smaller than other children and not able to do what others can, but to me, he is perfect in every way. We have already had our first visit with our special care clinic at the local children's hospital (and met many wonderful families who have walked the DMD journey before us. I was given a local woman's number who also has a son with DMD. I asked, "if you had one piece of advice to give a mom who just learned her son had DMD, what would it be?" Without hesitation she said, "Don't cry about tomorrow, simply enjoy today!" What wise words those have been for me to ponder. I have found a great deal of support, encouragement, and hope. We are determined to enjoy, no savor, every moment with our son. We delight in our days with him and set our attention on all we have to be thankful for. In all honestly, I am both humbled and honored that God would pick me to mother this sweet child and walk this journey with him. Despite DMD, I cannot help but say, "Daniel has been fearfully and wonderfully made!"

*Jeanette Wood*

# Andrew, 20 Months Old

## *He's here now, and he's happy*

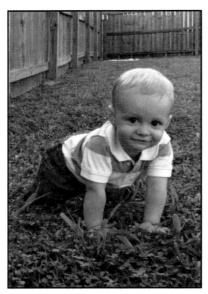

July Fourth weekend always starts off with a bang of some sort—the bang of a firework set off by the neighbors, the bang of the back door as your husband goes out to see if he has enough charcoal for the grill, or the bang of car doors slamming as the people around you head off for some Independence Day festivities. This past Fourth of July weekend did not start off with a bang for my family, it started with a ring. At 7:15 in the morning, my husband and I were awoken by a call on my cell phone. On the other end was my son's geneticist, and with his call came nine words that would strike fear in the heart of any parent: "How fast can you bring him into our ER?"

See, my then 18-month-old son, Andrew, was in his second month of specialists, tests, and procedures to try to find out why his gross motor skills were only at the level of a seven-month-old. Andrew wasn't crawling, pulling up, or even attempting to push himself into a seated position. We already had him enrolled in both physical and occupational therapy, but I knew there was something bigger than just low muscle tone going on with him. Thankfully, Andrew's pediatrician listened to my concerns and agreed that we should investigate why he was so weak. She referred us to a geneticist and a neurologist, which was how we arrived at the phone call at the beginning of the holiday weekend.

Andrew's creatine phosphokinase (CPK) level was off the charts and his liver enzymes were elevated. His geneticist was concerned about possible liver or kidney damage, hence the call to bring him in. So, with hearts pounding, my husband and I packed a bag, buckled Andrew into his car seat, and began the 45 minute drive to Vanderbilt Children's Hospital in Nashville. It was a near silent drive.

That weekend was a blur of needles, blood vials, scrubs, stethoscopes, consults, sleepless nights, and aching bones from pacing those concrete hospital floors. My heart broke with each needle that went into my sweet, innocent baby boy's body. He was practically a pin cushion for three days as one by one, tests were run and labs were sent out to make sure he was in no immediate danger.

During our final hours in the NICU, we were told that Andrew's blood would be sent out to Houston for a CPT II test, to Atlanta for a Duchenne/Becker test, and to the lab there at Vanderbilt for a myriad of other myopathic tests. It was then that it started to sink in with me that whatever was going on inside Andrew's tiny body to spike his CPK level so high was likely going to be a lifelong and possibly life-ending ordeal.

As I sat there feeling the fear of one day losing Andrew start to crush my heart, his attending physician came in to say goodbye before Andrew was discharged. She was very sweet, and I realized just how hard it must be on those doctors and nurses who become attached to these little angels who come into their NICU. Some leave there healthy and happy, some stay there their whole lives, and some leave there facing a whole new set of challenges. Andrew's attending physician talked with me for a bit about what a positive test for Duchenne/Becker would mean and how we should be thankful for the time we have with Andrew the way he is right now. Her parting words to me were, "He's here now, and he's happy." At first, I was a bit taken aback by her words. I didn't like what they implied. I tried to brush them off, but they never truly left my mind. I don't believe either of us realized the power that sentiment held or just how much those words would come to mean to me.

The first time the attending's words came back to me was after Andrew's geneticist called again. That time it was to tell us that Andrew did test positive for the Duchenne gene mutation, specifically, an out of frame deletion mutation of exon 45. The attending's words did not come back right away. Instead, I reacted much the same way as I believe any parent who is told their child has a fatal genetic flaw would react. My husband and I were devastated. There we were, totally in love with this child we created, and someone was telling us that one day we would no longer have him? It didn't seem right, didn't seem fair. It still doesn't. But after a few days of grief and prayer, those words surfaced in my mind and reminded me that what I have in Andrew this minute is a gift.

"He's here now, and he's happy". Of everything that anyone has said to me since learning that my baby is sick, this is what sticks out. That short sentence of encouragement and reality offered up from one of his NICU doctors has popped into my mind over and over again in the 10 weeks that I've known that my sweet Andrew has Duchenne Muscular Dystrophy. This doctor, whose name I don't even know, has single handedly yanked me back up off of the floor time and time again as her last sentence to me danced into the front of my mind from underneath the sorrow and grief DMD piled on top of it. "He's here now, and he's happy" reminds me that this little boy needs me to appreciate today. Andrew shouldn't be pulled down into despair with me; he should be delighting in the joys that today brings him. I shouldn't lie on the couch in pain. I should sit next to him on the kitchen floor and hand him Play-Doh. I should laugh alongside him as he squeezes it between his fingers and smashes it into his play mat. "He's here now, and he's happy" reminds me that right now is all any of us has. I cannot—I will not—spend what time I have with this beautiful boy drowning in the unjustness of what is to come.

In 1 Thessalonians 5:16-18, the Apostle Paul says to "Rejoice always, pray continually, give thanks in all circumstances; for this is God's will for you in Christ Jesus". He is reminding us that there is a reason bigger than ourselves for the events in our lives. God has a plan for each of us, and we are so blessed to have Him lighting our way. Even when the road is dark and bumpy, and veers off in a direction we had no intention of ever going, we should thank Him. We should thank Him for loving us enough to include us in His plan. I know that God chose ME to mother this child. He could have given me a genetically uncompromised child, but instead He chose me and my husband to care for one of His most precious souls, to do what others cannot. I do not ask, "Why us?" I say, "Why not us?" I know that God will not give us more than we can handle, and I believe that my husband and I can handle raising a child with Duchenne. This is not the life I had envisioned, but it is the life God envisioned for me, for my husband, and for my son. So I thank Him and I ask Him to guide me in the direction He wants me to go. I ask God to help me be the best mother possible for my Andrew. He picked me for this and I never want to let Him down. I never want to let my husband or my son down, either. That is precisely what I would be doing if I spent my time wallowing in the whys, the denials, or the despair of it all instead of celebrating the boy who is right in front of me. That is what the words, "He's here now, and he's happy" help me to do, stay present.

*Katherine Palmer*

## Aidan, 2 Years Old

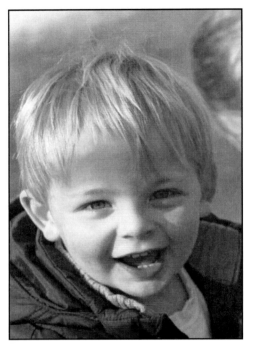

My husband, Stephen, and I have three children. Jacob is six, Abby is four, and Aidan is two. We welcomed Aidan into our home in April, 2010. He was six months old. He was healthy and had a smile on his face that could light up a room. He had a few delays due to being born prematurely. Also, his birth mother took drugs through her pregnancy. We knew he would have some issues but didn't think they would be anything like what he has to deal with.

In March, 2011, I got a call from Aidan's daycare that he had a high fever and wasn't feeling well. I picked him up and took him straight to the doctor. The doctor said he had some kind of infection and they would give him a shot of antibiotics and some Motrin. They said not to worry, that he would probably be sleepy and restless. We got home, and I put him in the crib to take a nap. About forty-five minutes later, I went to check on him to see if his fever was going down. When I went to his crib, I saw he was seizing. I picked him up, and as soon as I did, my mom called. I picked up the phone screaming and crying. She was in my driveway trying to get in the front door. I unlocked the door and she called 911. It felt like they were taking forever to get to my house. I didn't know what to do. He was my baby. Of course, you think to yourself, what did I do? Did I do this to him? Is he going to be okay?

The ambulance took Aidan and me to the hospital. He seized the whole way there. Doctors looked at him and gave him some medicine and took blood. After he got some IV fluid in him, he started to feel better and he perked up a little. They said he had a febrile seizure, which is common at his age, and he had a virus. They told us it would take some time for the virus to get out of his system. We took Aidan home and gave him fluids and medicine to keep his fever down. Every three and a half hours we got up and gave him medicine all through the night. The next morning he started throwing up. About 1:00 p.m., I told my husband that I could not do this anymore, that we were taking him to a children's hospital. His fever was still not going down and he couldn't keep anything down. We took him to an urgent care children's hospital. They ran blood tests and did chest x-rays. They said it was some kind infection but didn't know what. They tried to give him medicine and keep his fever down, but nothing worked. They transferred Aidan and me to the Children's Hospital of Atlanta. Aidan was admitted, and they had to do a spinal tap on him.

The doctors could not figure out what was going on. Aiden was in the hospital for about five days. He was feeling better, started to eat, and his fever finally went down to normal. They said it was probably a virus and they still were running tests, but we might never know what happened. They did tell us his liver enzymes were still elevated, but probably because of the virus. We would need to see someone in six weeks just to check his liver enzymes and make sure they were going down. We thought we were in the clear, but I just had a feeling something wasn't right. No one at daycare or in our home was sick. Aiden stayed home for another week with me to make sure his immune system was getting better. A couple of weeks passed, and we had an appointment to see a gastroenterologist. We went to the gastroenterologist, and he said that Aidan looked healthy. They would do blood tests to make sure everything was returning to normal, but he didn't think anything would come of it. The blood tests came back and his liver enzymes were still high. They had gone up since the hospital stay. I was scared. I didn't know why or how this had happened.

The doctor referred us to a liver specialist. We finally got an appointment with one who saw Aidan. The liver specialists looked Aidan over and couldn't believe that the child who had the blood test and Aidan were the same kid. They took more blood and said they would see what was going on and would call us. They called two days later. Aiden's liver enzymes were really high. They said to bring him in one more time and they would do more testing. I just kept thinking, how much more blood can they take from him? They told us some tests wouldn't be in for a week so we should just do what we normally do while we waited for the results.

When they took the blood, of course, I asked what they were looking for and what they were testing for. They always just give you a broad range, but I do know how to read a paper and I do have some medical knowledge. They were looking for cancer, hepatitis—any disease you can think of, they were testing for it. A lot of things were going through my mind. What if he has cancer or something else? What if they cannot figure it out altogether? The unknown was killing us.

The liver specialist called Aidan's primary physician. They were almost to the point of saying, "Okay, he has something wrong, but we don't know what it is, but his body is attacking the liver." They said they were consulting one more doctor and then they might have a diagnosis. They called and said they needed more blood to check just a few more things. The next day, I got a phone call saying that his CPK test was 20,000. Of course, I didn't wait for an appointment to start researching what this could mean or what that could mean. At that point, Aiden had been hospitalized for a week, had seen a gastroenterologist and a liver specialist, and then they wanted us to see a neurologist. I think the liver specialist knew we were getting exhausted by so many different doctors. They called me on a Friday in July and said that they would be admitting Aidan to the hospital on Monday. His liver enzymes were still high, his CPK levels were still high, and we wanted to get some consultations. I knew this was best for Aiden, but it about killed me inside. I had so much stuff on my mind. My husband still had to work, and I had two other kids at home.

We were in the hospital for about four days. Aidan had a skin, liver, and muscle biopsy. We saw all kinds of specialists. The good news was that Aidan's liver was fine. I was so glad. But the bad news was that they still didn't know what was going on. They said when the muscle biopsy came back, they would know for sure why his CPK was high. These were the longest weeks of my life. We got a call, and they said his tests came back but didn't show much. I was so frustrated. The liver specialist said I needed to make an appointment with a neurologist. In August, 2011, we went to the MDA in Atlanta, Georgia. I kind of already knew what Aiden had, but I knew I needed a confirmation. After we went in, the doctor looked over Aiden's lab tests and said he had Duchenne Muscular Dystrophy. They said they needed to do a blood DNA test to figure out what gene was missing, but he had Duchenne.

I didn't break down. My mom and my mother-in-law were with me. The doctor told me the diagnosis, but I don't think it really hit me until the social worker there came in and started to talk about the Make-A-Wish Foundation. I wanted to break down, but I didn't want Aidan to see me get upset. They took his blood and said we would have his results in a few weeks. The worst for me was to tell my husband his baby boy had Duchenne. It hit the family hard. All of us just didn't know what to say or how to say it. Everyone knew my husband and I were in pain. I had bad days after that. One day I was angry and the next I was just a wreck. I didn't know if I would ever come out of this sadness and hurt. It started out with more bad days verses good days. Now I am having more good days verses bad days. I had to learn that it was okay to cry and be angry. It was okay to not to be okay with it. If you ever met Aidan, you wouldn't know he has a disease. Duchenne doesn't define Aidan. Aidan is our strong, little boy. No matter what will come in our path, we will stand up as a family against it. People tell us that Aidan is lucky to have us as his parents, and I tell people that he isn't the lucky one; we are lucky to be his parents.

Stephen and I couldn't do what we do if it weren't for our parents. They have been our rock through this roller coaster of a year. Each day we cannot thank them enough for the love and courage they give us.

*Elaine Cabe*

## Connor, 4 Years Old

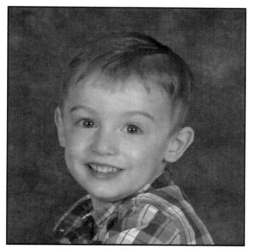

As I sit here and watch my wife cry, which seems to be a nightly occurrence, I wonder if there is anything I can do to help her. Do I love her? Yes. Do I feel badly? Yes. Am I sad? Yes. But all I know to do is to hug her and make sure everything in the house is done so she doesn't have to worry about "anything" other than work and Connor. For most women, moms, and parents, these painful emotions would be crippling, but my wife battles through them and continues on with her and Connor's daily routine, and that of our other three children, Liam, Declan and Keely. Me? I just make sure Connor and the other kids get everything they need: Love, hugs, OT, PT, meds, hydro therapy, daily stretches and regular doctor appointments. For Connor and others like him, there's so much more that goes along with this disease—a terrible, unforgiving disease.

As a certified Paramedic I have saved hundreds of lives. Some, in my mind, that did not deserve saving. That may sound harsh, but why is the drunk-driver-heroin-user the one that I can save but there is no training, miracle drug, blood transfusion or any other treatment that will save my son? That's right—my son. I constantly ask myself "why him?" "Why us?" "Why, why, why?" All of these why's, but very few answers. I know how Connor got it. I know what it is doing to His body. I know the treatment, and I also know that this disease will kill him before his time. I wish there was something I could do to make ALL of this easier. I know there are not many fathers out there that can say they are the primary care givers of their household, but I am one of them. I feel that I cannot cry or get sad, depressed, or drowned in thought, because with all of those emotions come chaos, disorganization, unrest, and turmoil. I cannot allow that to happen. I feel if any of these things happen, Connor will not get what we parents or the doctors believe he needs. I feel that all of the work and effort we put in now will keep my son on this earth longer.

I know that somewhere out there, in a rock, in a lab, or in a plant, there is a cure for this horrible disease. I just hope that it can be bottled and given to every child with this disease, including my son!

*Jon Mullaly*

I learned what Duchenne was when my son, Connor, was diagnosed a year ago. It catapulted me into a whole other world: a world of disability; a world of genetics, science, and fatality; a much more difficult world than I had known before.

Parents don't typically think about their children's mortality, so a diagnosis like this is more than devastating. We are still grieving. We grieve that Connor won't be able to do the things his brothers and sister are able to do. We grieve because we know that EVERYTHING will be harder for him. We know that he will have to come to terms with his own mortality when he understands what Duchenne is. We know that there will never be an answer to the question, "Why?". And we grieve when we remember what we thought our family would be like.

I remember very vividly when we were on our way to the hospital because Connor's CK levels were astronomically high. We had talked to Dr. Brundage, our Pediatrician, again because Connor's developmental delays hadn't improved and we wanted to rule out something neurological. We had just had a very traumatic year with my husband's testicular cancer diagnosis, chemotherapy, and remission as well as a new baby, so we had shelved our concerns for the time being. I looked behind my seat at Connor happily sitting in his car seat watching the traffic. He was very excited to be up past his bedtime, and I remember thinking to myself, *he doesn't look sick.* Surely he would look sick if something was wrong. The thought didn't make any sense to me since I knew that there can be unseen problems. There were certain pieces that didn't make any sense, which is why we were on our way to the hospital. His perpetual nose bleeds because he fell when learning to walk, which was late, which led to his nickname "The Nose Bleed Kid". Connor didn't crawl until after a year. He made most of his milestones, but they were at the very end of the spectrum. We thought his personality seemed to be a "watcher" since his speech was exceptionally delayed, but he was getting Early Intervention support already for speech. His balance, however, was never good, but not bad enough to qualify for support. But Connor always loved to dance—we have endless videos of Connor and his older brother "Raising the Roof". Nothing prepared us for Duchenne.

We had a hard time getting back from the hospital. I couldn't function at work: I cried all the time, including in front of the kids. The only thing I cared about was educating myself on Duchenne. How do I save my son? There must be some way, but everything I read had "fatal" plastered all over it. Who wouldn't trade places with their child out of desperation? At that time, Connor's favorite thing to do was dance. It got harder and harder to watch him because I kept thinking about how eventually; he wouldn't be able to do that anymore. We kept it up for a while, but also got worried about how much damage it was doing, so we stopped encouraging him to dance.

It's so hard when your three-year-old is looking into your eyes and you keep thinking *"he doesn't know"*.

We were lucky though. Dr. Brudage did the CK test that led us to Dr. Filiano, a pediatric neurologist who knew about Duchenne and what to look for. On Connor's discharge we were pretty sure he had Duchenne, but we needed to wait two weeks for the genetic test to come back. We have learned over the past year that our timeline for knowing Connor's diagnosis is a dream in comparison. It has made us appreciate the little things. We are also lucky that Connor is the only one in our family afflicted with Duchenne.

There is most definitely a *before* Duchenne and *after* Duchenne. While switching out photos around the house or looking at past memories, the very first thought is "Was that before or after?" We are early on in the journey of Duchenne, and we know that these feelings will diminish over time, but it's still quite fresh "only" a year into this.

Duchenne also introduced us to the world of disability. Before Connor's diagnosis, we were blissfully unaware of this "other world". All television ads applied to us; for example, the soccer mom letting all the kids pile out of the minivan at the park. She has no wheelchair ramp. Everything is tainted now because the world isn't designed for us, we know live in this "other world".

Needless to say, our world has changed dramatically. Our new greeting has changed to "What exon deletion is your son?" We have thrown ourselves into learning everything there is to know about DMD. We have said that we feel like we needed to become experts overnight about everything.

The Duchenne Community has been amazing; they are truly the only ones who "get it". Family and friends can sympathize, but only another family with Duchenne can empathize. Be sure to reach out to the support groups from MDA, the Parent Project Community site, and Facebook groups for Duchenne.

So we try to count our blessings and be more appreciative of the moment. And Connor has started dancing again.

*Kira Mullaly*

## Cooper, 4 Years Old

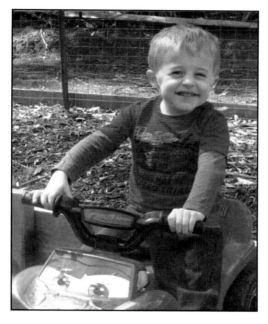

I had always heard of the expression, *Life can change in an instant*.

I never considered that I would ever experience this in my own life. Didn't this type of thing happen only in the movies? Well, that's what I thought until June 16, 2011. This date will be burned into our life story forever....

I am a wife and the mother of three beautiful children. It was all I ever dreamed of growing up. I always knew what I wanted in life. Looking back, I can now see that I had to work hard, persevere, and struggle to get all that I have achieved.

I wanted to have a career teaching children. I wanted to fall in love and I wanted to get married and have a healthy family...three kids in all. Surely it wasn't too much to ask for, was it?

I met Matthew, my husband, and together we had Mitchell, age five; Cooper, age four; and our daughter Reese, age 15 months. Mitchell had always achieved his milestones early and had a problem only with speech. Cooper, on the other hand, had always been a more relaxed and carefree child. So when he didn't crawl until 13 months and then walk at 19 months, it was not alarming to us, as that was just our Cooper. He was only one month outside the normal range of motor skill acquisition anyway. No problem.

Beginning when Cooper was about two and a half, friends and family began to remark about how 'lazy' he was. Requests to pack up toys, or hop up to the table for dinner or to catch up when walking were met with constant replies of, "Me can't mum!" "Me don't want to!" I thought this was surely the result of the terrible twos' behavior in another form. Don't I look back now with obvious regrets!

We would often giggle at Cooper as he would run. Cooper would pump his arms with effort, lifting his shoulders, but would still be walking. We all thought it was just so cute. But at age three and a half, his difficulties became alarmingly apparent when he was compared to his peers. Why did Cooper constantly play in the sandpit? Why couldn't he pedal a bicycle? Why could he make it to the toilet in time, but not be able to climb up with a step that assisted other children? Things just didn't seem right and day-by-day; those niggling doubts began to really bother me, until the bother became glaringly obvious: something was *just not right!* His swimming teacher brought to my attention that Cooper was lacking leg strength. He had considerable difficulty climbing out of the pool, unlike the other three-year-olds in his class.

The following week I had our scheduled appointment for Cooper's three-and-a-half-year-old check with the local health nurse. Our usual health nurse was not there. But the lady filling in listened to my concerns and her comment was, "Well, he can kick a ball across the room. He seems fine, but check with your doctor." That was the final straw. Blasé comments weren't enough anymore.

I met with my doctor later that day and explained my concerns. He was wonderful (and still is to this day). Initially, he dispelled all my fears when he said, "Donna, all kids develop differently. Don't compare him to Mitchell." I had a five-year-old and a three-and-a-half-year-old and a nine-month-old at that time. I was finding three young children challenging and I needed to relax. Surely, I just needed to relax! That's what everyone was telling me to do. Who was I to argue with professionals? That was in April.

But something inside just kept nagging at me. I was uneasy with the fact that Cooper would unsuccessfully try to pedal a bike. He *wanted* to ride, but he couldn't. He was not being lazy, as the desire was there. He was becoming increasingly frustrated with his inability. Surely, if he were lazy, he wouldn't care, he wouldn't be bothered. But he was also continuously falling (as all DMD parents would now be enlightened as to why), and he was sleeping for increasingly longer hours. Cooper would even disappear mid-afternoon and I would find him in his bed asleep. *Always tired, always falling, always frustrated!* It just didn't seem right. But I was told to relax and let it go. And I tried to—but it was always there.

A few weeks later, Cooper's most wonderful preschool teachers, Shar and Jo, asked if I would mind if they referred Cooper for an O.T. (occupational therapy) assessment. They had concerns that Cooper was having obvious physical difficulties keeping up with his peers. What surprised me later was my reaction. Not questioning, not denial, not disbelief, but an overwhelming sense of relief. Relief that someone else was confirming my concerns. That someone else was acknowledging…there was *SOMETHING WRONG!*

From that conversation, I went home and made the next available appointment with our family doctor. And the teachers and I began looking at exactly what Cooper's limitations were. His right leg could be straightened in the air but his left couldn't quite get there.

We decided, as we thought we were such experts now, that Cooper would probably just need some physiotherapy. But when I met with our doctor, I was going to request a hip x-ray to eliminate anything major like hip dysplasia. In the meantime, I had told Cooper, "We'll see the doctor. He'll give us some stretches; maybe physio, and then you'll be able to ride your bike." Oh, how I regret saying that to him now!

So we met with our doctor and I explained that now not only did I have concerns, but that Cooper's kinder teachers did, also. I explained that I knew I was probably being silly, but I would like Cooper's legs to be 'physically' examined and a hip x-ray ordered to rule out any major skeletal abnormalities. I was thinking worst case scenario, that Cooper may require surgery for some skeletal correction. Oh, if only!

Our doctor looked at Cooper's legs and agreed that there was an issue. He then ordered a bilateral hip x-ray. To receive our results, we had to return for those three days after the x-ray was taken. So with all three of my children, I marched next door to make an appointment. I think the look of dire concern and the three children age five and under may have created a sense of urgency, as we were led straight through to have the x-ray taken then and there. Three days later I was back in the doctor's office, where I was told the results were clear, and I was going to be referred to a pediatrician for further investigation. His guess was that it was possibly something neuro-muscular. So what does any nervous mother do when confronted with medical jargon? The only thing she can do when waiting over three weeks for the next appointment…GOOGLE!

So I started looking up neuromuscular. Just what exactly did neuromus-cular mean? And off I went.

"Oh look at that!" …*Children are late to walk (Cooper at 19 months) find it challenging to run, ride a bike, has a waddling gait and difficulty rising from the floor, a protruding belly and enlarged calves.* That was a perfect description of Cooper. "What was this called again?" I said to myself. "*Duchenne Muscular Dystrophy*…Du-what?" *Child requires the assistance of a wheelchair in mid-primary…* I remember thinking to myself' Oh, Donna, stop googling. You're being melodramatic again. Just wait for the professionals to investigate!" I no longer had a sense of urgency to research anymore. This was typically unlike me.

June 16, 2011, arrived and it was a day of devastating news for more rea-sons than one. At four a.m., I had been woken by a text message from a girlfriend to tell me her son, Noah, who was a friend of my eldest son, Mitchell, had been diagnosed with Leukaemia two days earlier. He was currently in hospital receiving chemo. My heart went out, offering anything I could do to assist her.

My mother had come to look after Mitchell and Reese while I took Cooper to see the pediatrician for his consultation. I remember hearing a lady before me complaining quite loudly. I was thinking that at least we would be a quick and easy patient. A bit of physio and we'd be fine. How wrong was I?

The paediatrician examined Cooper. "Big calves," he commented. "That's important." He asked Cooper to get up off the floor. "Gower's sign! Hmmm that's important!" I remember thinking; does he want me to take notes? I sat down as he was gathering his thoughts and he announced, "There is a problem. I believe it is a muscular dystrophy, most likely Duchenne!"

It is a muscular dystrophy, most likely Duchenne!"

"Yep, ok."

The doctor looked at me and asked if I knew about it, and I replied very innocently, "Yes". But I didn't really. All I could say was, "Is that the one with the chair?"

He said "Yes." He explained I needed to get a blood test done that evening and, since it was 4:30 p.m., I had 90 minutes to get his blood test done somewhere. A follow-up appointment was squashed in for the following Monday afternoon. The doctor said that he would call me the next day with the blood test results. Matthew called me in the car to ask how the appointment went. I had a car full of kids and I couldn't explain as I had to keep myself together. He was driving nearby and I asked him to meet me in the car park in front of pathology. I left the kids in the car with my mum and ran to meet him. All the while I was thinking about how I would explain to Matt that our son might have Muscular Dystrophy and still hold myself together. I basically explained that the blood test would confirm the pediatrician's diagnosis and what that would mean for our Cooper. I could see everything in his eyes: pain, denial, disbelief and confusion. I felt helpless, as I could do nothing to help him. It wasn't the nicest way or the best place to be told such news.

Shortly after, we walked into the closest pathology department with Cooper. But the nurses there said that they were unable to take blood from children after 12 noon, as they needed the assistance of another nurse. So we had to get back into our cars and race to the nearest hospital. My mum stayed in the car park with Mitchell and Reese while Matthew, Cooper, and I stepped into our new life…hospitals and hand holding. Holding Cooper's hand, holding each other's hands, or simply holding my hands together and praying for this to be just a nightmare.

As Matthew started deliberating possible misdiagnosis, I became comfortable with the fact that I didn't need a blood test to confirm it. I knew inside that the diagnosis explained it. All the symptoms made sense. They had described Cooper's life exactly.

As I was driving everyone home, I was thinking, so my son is going to be a paralympian! That's ok. One of my friends had an accident playing Aussie Rules football and is now an Australian paralympian. The goal posts had shifted, but as a teacher, I was automatically gathering resources to reshift the goals. I'd introduce Cooper to my friend and that would give Cooper a focus. All good, I could do this!

It wasn't until we were all home that Matthew questioned something I hadn't thought of. "What about Cooper's life expectancy?"

I remember saying, "Cooper has weak muscles. That's all. He'll just need a wheelchair." But I, too, could no longer avoid it. The question was out there now, and I needed to know. So the computer went on (I can hear the collective sigh as you read this)…and I Googled, *Duchenne Muscular Dystrophy Life Expectancy…*

The results were up. The MDA (Muscular Dystrophy Association) stated, "Boys with Duchenne are expected to live into their 20's"

What happened next I had seen in the movies but never thought it would happen to me. But sure enough, as I was reading the facts on the screen, my legs went from under me and Matt caught me in sobs before I fell on the floor. "My baby, my precious baby boy, no not my baby…this can't be happening!" We were beyond distraught. I could never understand people who complained of being unable to sleep with worry, as I have always been the heaviest and best sleeper. But that night I understood. I am unsure if Matthew and I got even two hours of sleep. In the morning, we waited. Matt doubted what I had told him. And why not? He hadn't heard it himself. He hadn't seen the sadness in the doctor's face as he was telling me.

But the phone call came just after lunch. Our pediatrician called to say that Cooper's blood test results for the leaking enzyme, Creatine Phosphokinase, was 30,138. Most people without muscular dystrophy have a count of less than 240 units. So the reality was there. The results confirmed that my baby boy had a genetic disorder, *Duchenne Muscular Dystrophy*. We were then referred to the neuromuscular clinic at the Royal children's hospital. Our pediatrician had actually spoken to the Associate professors at the clinic, which sped up the process.

Follow-up DNA testing has shown that I am a carrier of the Duchenne Muscular Dystrophy gene. My mum was cleared as not having the mutation. My then pregnant sister was cleared as well. So I can often be heard jokingly saying to Mum, "I always said I was special and here's the proof!" But I don't think she's recovered her sense of humor at this stage.

Many people say to me, "Donna you shouldn't feel guilty; you can't blame yourself." No, I don't feel guilty, as I did not do this to Cooper intentionally. However, as a mother, you do feel a sense of responsibility. He is my son, I passed on this gene, and it will change his life forever. But the same can be said for all the other genes that Matthew and I passed on, like his cheeky sense of humor, his dad's good looks and, of course, I'd like to think, my empathy and compassion that he shows every day.

Dealing with this has its ups and downs. I laugh and smile more; I try to complain less. Grief comes hard and fast for the smallest instances, but subsides just as quickly. For example, when watching Cooper laugh as he runs from waves at the beach trying to catch him, I start sobbing instantly, but I need to quickly compose myself so as not to ruin his experience.

I am blessed to have the family and friends that I have, and I would not wish to change anything. Except maybe the deletion of exon 12 of the Dystrophin Gene. But that's not to be!

In talking with my cousin Paul recently, his wise words were, "You will now truly experience life. You will live all extremes of emotions. You will see beauty in the smallest details!" And I do, every day.

*Donna Anderton*

# Liam, 4 ½ Years Old

## Bits and Pieces, Bits and Pieces

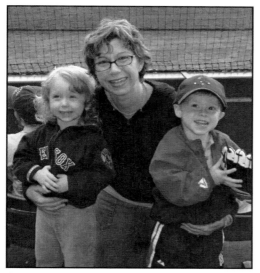

People important to you, people unimportant to you, cross your life, touch it with love and carelessness and move on. There are some people who leave you and you breathe a sigh of relief and wonder why you ever came into contact with them. There are people who leave you and you breathe a sigh of remorse and wonder why they had to go away leaving such a gaping hole. Children leave parents, friends leave friends, and acquaintances move on, people change houses, people grow apart. Enemies hate and move on. Friends love and move on. You think of the many that have moved into your hazy memory. You think of those present and wonder.

*"I believe in a master plan in life, people moving in and out of each other's lives and each leaves a mark on the other. You find you are made up of bits and pieces of all who ever touched your life and you are more because of it, and you would be less if they had not touched you. I hope you accept the bits and pieces with humility and wonder, and never question and never regret."*

*Bits and Pieces –Lois Cheney*

For the past two years I have been on an emotional roller coaster. I have experienced all the emotions of the grieving process: denial, anger, guilt, depression and acceptance. When people have asked me how I'm doing, the

*49*

words have been hard to find. This summer I participated in my first sprint triathlon. I was part of an incredible group of 85 women called the "Gals for Cal". I was joined by family, friends, and 8 other moms with sons who are affected by Duchenne Muscular Dystrophy (DMD). We swam, biked and ran to raise awareness and money for DMD. Our group was asked to speak at the Expo the day before the race to talk about why we "TRI". Nancy Halter Glendinning, co-founder of the Gals, started by saying. "When a child is diagnosed with Duchenne Muscular Dystrophy it takes his parents' breath away."

I feel like my breath has been taken away, and I grapple every day with the challenge of trying to catch my breath and go on with life.

Liam is the first born of my two children. He came peacefully into this world at 6:20am on the first day of spring in 2007. Unlike some families affected by DMD. We did not suspect anything was wrong with him. The only possible red flag was that he walked late at 19 months. His diagnosis of DMD was an incidental finding. Liam was 2 ½ years old when we decided to have his small stature worked up. Up until that time he had barely been on the growth chart. It was no big deal, a little blood work and a hand x-ray. Everything was normal except his liver enzymes were a little elevated, most likely due to a virus. When we repeated the labs a few weeks later and they were still elevated, we were sent to the Liver Clinic at Boston Children's Hospital. Further blood work revealed that Liam's Creatinine Kinase, which indicates muscle wasting, was 19,000. The normal range is in the 200s. Genetic testing confirmed DMD, a muscle wasting disease that affects all major muscles. The facts of DMD are daunting; most boys are wheelchair bound by the age of 12, their heart and lungs are affected in their teen years, and they don't often live beyond their 20's. Our lives have never been the same; our breath has been taken away.

Liam is an old soul at the tender age of 4 ½. He is always thinking of his little sister Abby and wants to make sure to include her. He loves trains, cars, baseball, and fire engines. He never forgets anything, but he already knows that things are more challenging for him than his peers. He takes daily steroids that we get from the United Kingdom because they have fewer side effects than those available in the United States. He takes daily medicine that will hopefully protect his heart from cardiomyopathy, which takes the lives of many young men with DMD. He goes to weekly physical and occupational therapy to increase his strength, flexibility, and endurance. He wears braces when he sleeps to keep his heel cords stretched. His care is coordinated at the Massachusetts General Pediatric Neuromuscular Clinic. This family centered clinic allows us to see all of Liam's specialists on the same day and coordinates care between pediatric and adult specialists to help improve the long term outcomes for the children and families they care for.

From the outside Liam looks like any other 4 ½ year old. You would never know that his body is being affected by this fatal disease. One evening, after a long day, we stopped to pick up a pizza. Liam, Abby and I were waiting in line to pick up our order when Liam fell flat on his face. There was blood everywhere. I was right next to him. He was not horsing around, he had just gone to take a step forward. The stares of unbelief tore at my heart. I felt like such a bad mother. All I wanted to do was scream, "He has Duchenne Muscular Dystrophy. He will be wheelchair bound by the age of 12 and I will most likely outlive him." This is a part of everyday life for me and other families who are affected by this disease. You are so careful to avoid the ice, the uneven ground, the high curb, and then your son falls flat on his face on even ground standing right beside you.

I have hope and faith in God, science, and research, but I am also a realist. I know that if things don't change soon I will watch Liam's body fail before my eyes. I hope that Grammie Mary, Liam's great grandmother is right. She believes that Liam may be dependent on a wheelchair to help him get around someday, but will otherwise live a long happy life. A life where his disease does not impede any of his goals or dreams. I swim, bike and run for all the boys with DMD who can't. When I am tired and hot I think of Liam and try my hardest not to stop. My husband and I have started a foundation called Liam's L.E.E.P. We coordinate and take part in fundraisers to increase awareness and raise funds to make Grammie Mary's dream come true. I hope that by the time Abby is thinking about becoming a mother that DMD is a disease of the past.

I believe in a master plan that God does not give us more than we can handle. I think of all the wonderful people in our lives because of Liam and Duchenne and I strive to "accept the bits and pieces with humility and wonder, and never question and never regret."

*Kristen McGourty*

# Chase, 4 Years Old

## Our Beautiful Son

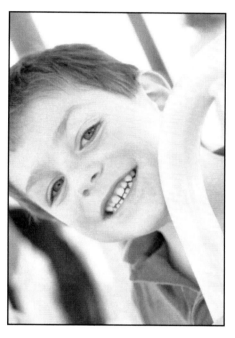

We are very new to the Duchenne community. Our son, Chase, is four years old. He is a happy and sweet-natured little boy who loves to snuggle. He was diagnosed with Duchenne Muscular Dystrophy in August of 2010. He was also diagnosed with moderate to severe autism with severe developmental delays in December of 2009. It was a long and frustrating road for a few years before finally getting to a diagnosis for either one. When Chase was born, he was alert, happy, and healthy and loved to eat. He grew so fast and was always above average on all his checkups. Height and weight were always above 97 percentile. He had great eye contact and was initiating peek-a-boo on his own at five months.

## Chase Was Noticeably Different From His Peers

Then at about a year old, we started to notice some things about Chase that concerned us. Why wasn't he trying to walk yet? Shouldn't he be saying at least mama or dada? Why wouldn't he look at most people anymore? Why was he such a picky eater? Why was he so noisy? I had also noticed that he seemed to be getting sick, A LOT. It seemed that every month for the previous three months he had gotten sick, not with a cold that lasted for a few days, but one that lasted for three weeks. I brought up my concerns with his pediatrician at the time. She said not to worry, that he was probably a little slow and not to compare him to my daughter because boys are slower than girls. This went on the same way for another three to four months. Chase was still getting sick every month and couldn't kick the illness without antibiotics. He was still not uttering a word, only making noises that seemed to be getting louder as time passed. Still not even one step taken, and he seemed to be getting clumsier.

## My Endless Search For Answers Begins

I started to search the Internet, typing in all the concerns I had. I even came across Muscular Dystrophy in my search. I asked our pediatrician and another one (in the same office) about MD. One said it was genetic and not to worry if it's not in your family. The other said that Chase was too strong and healthy, that if he had MD he would be more frail and weak. So I dropped it and started to search other areas, autism being one of them. The pediatrician did not seem to be listening to my concerns with the exception of the speech. She said we should get his hearing checked so I went to get a conventional hearing test. Chase did not cooperate, so they wanted another test. This time they would sedate Chase, but he needed a physical first. With the physical came an abnormal blood test, with elevated liver enzymes. We went to a pediatric GI doctor who ran a zillion blood tests, came up with nothing, and just monitored the liver enzyme levels for a few months. Still no change, so he wanted a liver biopsy. That came back fine.

Finally, I was sick of it. I got a new pediatrician, and he knew right away that Chase needed therapy. He ordered speech and occupational therapy to start immediately. But there was still no decline in liver enzymes. We also did the hearing test, Cystic Fibrosis testing, a swallow study, ultrasounds, x-rays. The GI doctor wanted to monitor for another year and then have another liver biopsy if there was still no reduction. I was not going to wait a year!

## *The Final Push To Get To The Bottom Of It All*

I was referred to a new GI doctor at Phoenix Children's Hospital, and she seemed to know the problem immediately. She ordered a CK test and that confirmed her suspicions, but we still needed to do more testing. In the few months that we had to wait for the appointment with the neurologist, I researched the heck out of neuromuscular disease. By the time we got there, I was pretty well informed on DMD, but I didn't give up hope that it was maybe a less severe form of MD. We saw the neurologist, and he gave a diagnosis of DMD before the genetic test was done. We sent it on and got the confirmation that it was, in fact, right there in black and white, proof that Chase did have this dreadful thing called Duchenne. Our world turned upside down and nothing was the same. With the autism diagnosis, I was sad for Chase, but it wasn't the same. Autism wasn't going to result in my son's passing away before he even had the chance to become a man, fall in love, or have children of his own. The pain was so bad, as if he had already been taken from us. The next several months were not really any better. We went to an MDA meeting thinking maybe the support group thing may help. Well, we were only a month in, and that was way too much for us to handle. With the exception of meeting some pretty amazing parents that had boys like Chase, we left the meeting feeling worse about Duchenne than before we got there! We both cried the entire hour plus drive home. All we could do was embrace him and keep him close and try to fake the fact that we were completely heartbroken.

## *The Lack Of Family Support Was Overwhelming*

When family members found out, a few called and said to call if we needed anything. Some were in utter denial (just as they were about the autism) and chose to be completely ignorant about it. Most of them never said a word, no call no nothing until they saw us at Thanksgiving and Christmas. Then it was, "Awww, poor Chase"! We were surprised at the lack of emotion and support from certain family members. It makes me so sad because Chase is such a wonderful little person with lots of love to give. With or without Duchenne and autism, he is so amazing and brings light into the hearts of everyone who meets him. It was especially hard for me because none of my family is in Arizona, and I didn't have them close by for support.

### Getting It Together and Becoming a
### True Advocate for Chase and All of 'Our' Sons

We soon created "Chase for the Cure," our group name for the MDA walk. We raised just short of $10,000 in a few months. During the walk, I had to focus on not crying. It was a very humbling experience seeing all of those young people in wheelchairs. It really makes you appreciate what you have. But I kept seeing Chase in those wheelchairs. It was really hard to imagine it because he is so full of energy and is constantly running circles around us. I get tired just watching him sometimes. My husband and I were both in a dark place for a while. We stopped going to the gym, started eating out a lot, and didn't want to do much at all. I gained about 25 pounds and didn't even care. We both realized that we needed to get it together and focus. What good were we to Chase if we stayed in that frame of mind? And when we realized that there was no family support here in Arizona, it was a huge wakeup call. We went to a few Duchenne events and met some pretty great parents of DMD children. We even got together with a few parents on our side of town and formed a group that meets once a month.

I have been getting better at dealing with my feelings and finding ways to redirect myself for the better. Don't ever be afraid of questioning your doctor if you feel that there is a lack of knowledge or urgency. You are the only advocate for your child. If I hadn't pushed so hard for my doctors to make a move, I still would not have a diagnosis for Chase. All I can tell a parent with a new DMD diagnosis is this: cherish every moment with your children and love and laugh often with them. All you can do is live life like the next breath is your last. Never give up hope because we WILL find a cure!

*Seavey Castelli*

## Jonah, 7 and Emory, 5 Years Old

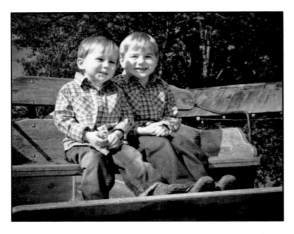

It was a week before Christmas in 2008, and I was on the way from Dickson, Tennessee, to Arkansas to see customers. I had made it to Memphis when my wife called and asked if I could pull off the road, at which time I couldn't. Then she asked, "Do you see an exit?" Again I couldn't stop, but I told her, "Whatever it is, just tell me."

She then said it was about Jonah, our oldest son, who at the time was five. He had been to the pediatrician's office that day to get all of his shots for kindergarten. The doctor called Sonya out of the office, which is where she works as a pediatric nurse. Dr. Betts told her he thought Jonah had muscular dystrophy because of his enlarged calf muscles. At that point I had pulled off the road and Sonya told me that I needed to come home because the next day they wanted to test Emory. Since the type of MD they thought Jonah had was genetic, Emory could also have it.

We took Emory to the pediatrician's office for testing. Then we went to see the neurologist while they were getting the test results back from the lab. While we were in the consultation with the neurologist, the nurse told Sonya that she had a call. It was the news that I never thought we could possibly receive. Emory's blood test came back positive, so they both had MD. Our next step was to get the chromosome test to see which form of MD they had. We found out they both had Duchenne Muscular Dystrophy.

That Christmas was the most meaningful Christmas I ever remember having because it wasn't about the presents, it was about cherishing the time together that for so long we had taken for granted. Our boys were only five and two, so they had no idea how all of our lives would be changed forever. It was a time that, no matter what happened, nothing else seem to matter because our perspective on life was completely different. I own a small manufacturing company, and three weeks after my sons' diagnoses, one of my biggest automotive customers filed bankruptcy and left us with over $150,000 worth of invoices we would never receive payment for. It didn't affect me because the most important thing wasn't work or money. It was appreciating life and the blessings that God gave our family.

Over the next year, we went to a lot of doctor's appointments and did even more research on DMD. We live in Middle Tennessee and saw the doctors at Vanderbilt Children's Hospital. But we also went to Washington, D.C., to see Dr. Hoffman at Children's National. We wanted to go to D.C. because we knew Dr. Hoffman named the dystrophin gene that causes all the problems with Duchenne kids. We were still in the fog about diagnosis but wanted our boys to know why they couldn't run or keep up with the other kids their age. We set Jonah and Emory down to tell them that they had Duchenne Muscular Dystrophy and that one day they would have to be in a wheelchair. Jonah looked at us and said, "Cool. I will need two of them, a fast one and a slow one, so when I am in my slow one my friends can keep up with me."

When the fog of diagnosis lifted and we started seeing the cruel signs of DMD, like when our boys started struggling going up steps, it just broke our hearts. We decided at that point we wanted to do more, so we started FightDMD.com to fund research for Duchenne Muscular Dystrophy. The Duchenne families are faced with two huge obstacles, which are time and money. I don't want our sons to have limits in life, so we are aggressively fundraising so one day a cure will be found.

In the second year of diagnosis, we started yearly cardiologist visits with Dr. Markham, which I would recommend to all Duchenne parents, because we found our youngest son had an enlarged heart. Our boys have the same disease with the same exon deletions but show different symptoms of this disease. Jonah's heart is completely normal, and at this point, we have controlled, with heart medicine, our youngest son's heart enlargement. We all know the statistic that 75% of Duchenne patients lose the battle against DMD because of heart failure. If we had waited to see a cardiologist, our current success of controlling Emory's heart could have been completely different.

We are currently in the third year of this horrible disease, and even though it's not getting easier on our kids, we still have hope a cure will be found in time for this generation of Duchenne boys. It would not be possible to stay positive without the many thoughts, prayers and generous gifts that our friends and family in Middle Tennessee have given us. To date we have raised over $110,000 for Duchenne research, but we couldn't have done it alone, so thank you to all those that have supported our family.

FightDMD.com has been established since April of 2010 and we have hosted 2 golf tournaments, a celebrity basketball game and a half marathon. We have covered Tennessee by hosting a tailgate fundraiser at UT Knoxville in East TN, several events in our hometown of Dickson and a 5k run at UT Martin in West TN. The local high school supported us by having a soccer game and donating all the proceeds from the gate to our foundation and our family has had several bake sales.

Jonah played on a baseball team in the summer of 2011 and had to play most of the year with cast on both legs from the knee down. His feet were already contracting to the point we were discussing heal cord surgery to correct but luckily the cast worked temporarily. He played on a 7-8 year-old team and the other boys were inspired by his attempt to get out and continue to play even though he couldn't run like the other kids or bend down to get the ball if it came to him. At the end of the year one of the teams joined together and wanted him to get a home run so they inconspicuously threw the ball around until he made it to home plate at which time the umpire gave him the home run ball. All the fans on both sides were standing up cheering for him and when he walked by his mom he said "What did we win or something". Keep in mind these are 7 and 8 year old boys that came up with this idea.

Then the most rewarding event took place when the all-star team was chosen. The boys wanted to do more than allow Jonah to get a home run, so they started selling lime green arm bands with FightDMD and All-Stars for Duchenne on the armband. Within the first week the all-star team sold almost 2,000 armbands and made Jonah an honorary teammate. At the first game of the district tournament the league had Jonah throw out the first pitch. The boys were very talented and made it all the way to the World Series in South Carolina. This allowed them to raise more than $3,800 in armband sales. When we started FightDMD it was about raising the $500,000 as fast as possible, but in the short time since then, we have learned so much about life and enjoying each day like there is no tomorrow.

*Terry Marlin, Founder FightDMD*

# Jack, 5 Years Old

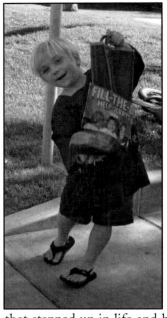

You don't know Jack? You Should!

First off, we, Jack's family, would like to thank you for reading our story.

Jack Robert Anderson was born on February 5ᵗʰ, 2006. It was Super Bowl week-end and the Seattle Seahawks were facing the Pittsburgh Steelers.

Who knew that he would be a *Blue Eyed* Angel with dimples that just invite you to take a second look? And when you take that second look, your heart is his **forever**. You, like Jack himself, will start referring to him as Jack Jack. He is named after three great men. His first name, Jack, is in honor of his great grandfather, John (who went by Jack). John was a man that stepped up in life and helped a lot of people out. He made a big impact on his grandson, Jeremiah, Jack Jack's dad. His middle name Robert is after his grandfather Floyd Robert. Floyd is a man that will do what it takes to get things done, and done right. His last name, Anderson, should read, "Its All Good Anderson" because Jack Jack's dad, Jeremiah, has a gift of seeing the good in every situation. This is a trait that he is passing on to his children.

Now that you know a bit of his heritage, let me tell you a little about Jack Jack. He is five years old. He is going to be the first firefighter dolphin trainer that trains Shamu after he completes a short stint in the Army. Jack Jack does not care much for television or video games. What he does like is to play with "his guys". You can play with Jack Jack and his guys (as long as it's the guy Jack gives you). Jack Jack's favorite thing to do is to go in his great grandpa Red's Jacuzzi in his boxers. Yup, I said boxers. Jack Jack has a big Brother Jacob, age 8. Their favorite family activity is the annual Renish/Hickey family reunion held every year during Memorial Day Weekend. This gathering allows for the entire family—somewhere around one hundred people—to camp with one another, to spend time together, and catch up on what happened in the past year. Jack Jack loves playing with his many cousins, and they love their time with him as well.

This little boy's life is being threatened by Duchenne Muscular Dystrophy (DMD). It is an inherited genetic disorder that affects mostly boys. DMD is a progressive disease that weakens and wastes the muscles of a boy's body, and causes respiratory and/or cardiac complications.

Jack's Family is committed to increasing the awareness of Duchenne Muscular Dystrophy, and raising money for research to develop new treatments and to find a cure. You can help us by checking out CUREDUCHENNE.ORG

*Lindy Wilhelm & Sarah Renish*

## Andrew, 5 Years Old

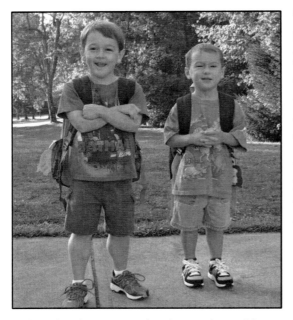

This is the story of two boys—one who has Duchenne and another who does not. When faced with a disease that will eventually take the life of your little boy, you have so many questions floating around in your head. Many of them, unfortunately, begin with why? Then there are the "how" questions, the ones that day after day we continually ask ourselves. How are we going to be able to be the parents that he needs, and how are we going to be able to also be parents to his little brother? How am I going to be that mommy that they both so desperately need?

You see, I'm not really different from any other moms who have dreams for their children. My dreams just seemed to have been shattered right before my eyes in September of 2009. That is when we first learned of Andrew's diagnosis. He was three years old. That is the day that will forever be engraved in my mind. Memories of those first precious weeks and months of his life came rushing back to me as we received the dreadful news. We had so many hopes and dreams for our boy and we wanted, most of all, for him to be happy. I felt that with a diagnosis of DMD, his future was over, done, gone. No college, no career, no wife, no kids, no grandkids and, most of all, no happiness.

As the days went on and those big brown eyes looked at me, and his little toddler grin continued to melt my heart, I knew that I was wrong. You see, also in the year 2009 we almost lost our youngest son, Ethan. It was April, 2009. He was 15 months old and in the Pediatric ICU fighting a horrible case of MRSA pneumonia. He was literally fighting for his life, and I felt right then and there the future of my precious boy was over. Then one night as I sat next to that awful white metal crib, praying to God to please, please not let him die, I realized that I had to let go and let God take care of the gift He had given me—that no matter how hard I wished or tried or thought I was in control, I absolutely was not. Then the most amazing peace came over me, and I awoke to a nurse telling me that Ethan's chest tube had fallen out on its own. Early the next morning, a team of doctors was standing over him with amazement in their faces. One of the doctors looked over at me and then to him and said, "I really don't know how he is still here with us." He shook his head a couple times and said again, "I really don't know." But I knew. And that day he began to miraculously recover and was able to leave the hospital two days later! God's purpose for Ethan was not yet fulfilled; he still needed to be here with us on this earth. Then five months later when I felt that I knew when the end of Andrew's life was going to be, I remembered that, no, I really didn't. Just like all the rest of us, his days are numbered, and only God knows how many he has. And when Andrew does reach heaven, he will be smiling down on us with those adorable dimples and big brown eyes. And the most awesome thing of all is that he will be running, running like the wind, running as he has never run before. He will be experiencing that happiness that we wished for him always and forever.

So right now I am going to enjoy these days of dog bones flushed downed the toilet, permanent marker stripes drawn on the countertop, Mommy's blush brush doused in Vaseline, shampoo squirted down the laundry chute for Batman "cause it makes him go faster" flour all over the kitchen because they want it to snow, sloppy ice cream kisses, jumping in big leaf piles, big bear hugs, and the list goes on and on. My boys and my God have taught me—have taught us—that we have to make a conscious choice that nothing in this life can take away our hopes and dreams for a future, absolutely nothing. We can either sit around and sulk, or we can get up, enjoy our life, love God, and live every moment as if it is the very last!

> "For I know the plans I have for you," declares the Lord, "plans to prosper you and not to harm you, plans to give you hope and a future." Jeremiah 29:11

*Jodi Heisey Nichols*

## Colin, 7 Years Old

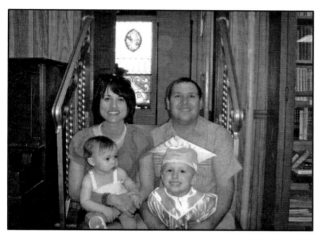

"You want to know what's wrong with your kid? I'll tell you what is wrong with your kid. It's Muscular Dystrophy and it's probably Duchenne." Can you believe these were the words of a neurologist? A professional person! My husband, John, and I set up an appointment with this doctor to determine why our son Colin could not jump & struggled climbing stairs. Colin was just 5 weeks shy of his 5th birthday. There probably is not a good way to hear this kind of news but if there is a possible worst way to hear it, we certainly experienced that!

At that time on June 26, 2009, my husband and I had an awareness of Duchenne Muscular Dystrophy. I worked with a little boy with Duchenne and he passed away at the age of 7 from heart complications. I had just a little more knowledge of the neuromuscular disease than John did at the time. So when the neurologist threw us overboard into the Arctic Ocean, John knew it was bad but did not know it was fatal. The good news is that John was able to keep himself together & listen to the neurologist's instructions on our next step which was to confirm this diagnosis. I, on the other hand, sat there sinking into a pit of despair. I sat there looking at my beautiful little boy thinking he will be dead in 2 years. Not only that but we will WATCH him slowly lose all of the skills he had developed to this point. At that point I could not hear anything the neurologist was saying. In fact all of the color began to drain from the room and I lost my peripheral vision. I sat there looking at my son in a world of black and shades of gray. Looking back I think my body went into protective mode. It began to feel like an out of body experience and I was sinking away from everyone & everything in the room. I came out of it as we were walking downstairs in the hospital. John explained that Colin had to have something called a CK test done. Whatever that meant! Something about muscle damage and CK leaking into the bloodstream.

After the test I picked up Colin and had this urge to run far away from this horrible thing called Duchenne Muscular Dystrophy. As if you could run away from a ball attached to your ankle by a chain. This disease was ravaging my son's muscles from the inside but I wanted to outrun it and hide Colin from this fate! So my tunnel vision and the shades of black and gray returned as I ran from that hospital with Colin in my arms.

When we returned home later that morning, we waited. The neurologist was to call us with the results of the creatine kinase test. About noon we received his call. I was told Colin's CK level was something like 24,000. The doctor then proceeded to tell us he would set up genetic testing then we would start "prednizone" the next month since Colin was 5 and you need to start steroids at the age of 5". I had to wrap my mind around this unbelievably high CK level. So when I asked again about the normal CK levels and repeated for my own unbelieving ears that his was 24,000, the doctor coldly corrected me and said, "No its 24,568" As if that additional 568 made one bit of difference! One thing I couldn't help notice was how proud this neurologist seemed to be that he was the one who was able to pinpoint exactly why Colin struggled with gross motor skills. He appeared so focused on that fact and got busy planning his next move that he totally lost sight of the fact that he devastated a family in the process. The next words out of my mouth were, "I need a second opinion." He said, "No one will be able to tell you anything different. In fact if they tell you there is going to be a cure, they will be misleading you. When there is a cure, it will be broadcast on every media outlet possible. Right now don't think 2 years into the future (there's that 2 years again!) just enjoy your time with your son." I hung up and began to have a panic attack. I had this weight in the center of my chest that would not let me breathe. I just hoped that there was some doctor out there who could show us compassion by acknowledging the fact that our life took a lonely detour. Most people walk down life's path smiling and we were thrown off that path into a ditch.

Just a few weeks prior to the neurologist appointment we had Colin evaluated by the early intervention program within our local intermediate unit. After nearly a year of the pediatrician telling us Colin was just slightly delayed in gross motor skills we decided to push for more help. We started private PT but after 2 months of treatment insurance denied any more visits. At that time, Colin was only diagnosed with a developmental delay. Our private PT stated that she did not see signs of a progressive disease.

This is when, what I call our God moments began. I have personally experienced amazing signs of God's love and presence that have helped me and my whole family survive. I do not want to alienate you, the reader, by telling you about my experiences if you have not had such events happen to you. My goal is to offer you comfort. Whatever your religious beliefs may be, I want to tell this story to show you that there is a higher power looking out for each one of us to offer comfort and gentle guidance. Families slapped by Duchenne are given a bittersweet gift. I don't say touched because there is nothing gentle about this disease. On one hand you are crushed by the sheer weight of what Duchenne MD means. But on the other, you are shown a side of life you may never have experienced had you never heard of the disease before.

The day after the unofficial diagnosis, I called my pastor and cried out my pain to his voicemail from the floor of my bathroom. I didn't sleep much that night and spent most of it either sitting on the couch with John or lying next to Colin holding him tightly! John's parents are our neighbors and our kids love walking over to Mommom and Poppop's house to visit. My in-laws invited us over for lunch the next day. My husband walked over with the kids for lunch and I stayed home sitting on the porch swing. My pastor returned my call and we prayed together over the phone. Then it hit me when I realized I never really prayed before. Sure I had been raised with faith, attended Sunday school as well as Bible school and went to church. But I never really knew how to pray. I sat there looking up at the sky watching the clouds go by thinking about that fact. Then I saw an odd cloud shape come into view. It had a defined head with a long flowing body as if covered in a robe and two distinct wings outstretched. Immediately, John's grandmother came to mind. She had passed away in 2008 when I was pregnant with our daughter Sara. So being a bit skeptical, I kept looking at the sky thinking did I just see that? Then the second cloud shape came into view. It was bigger than the first, again with a defined head, a body covered in a robe and two outstretched wings that reached down towards me. Now my Grandfather came to mind. He passed away in 2002 just after John and I were married. I kept thinking what did I just see? Then I said my first kind of prayer, "If it is you two, please help me. We have a doctor that has zero compassion and we need a new one. Please help me find a doctor who will give us hope. Then I sat there trying to see if I saw any more angel clouds. My husband came in and interrupted me with a plate of food. So I sat down in the kitchen and the phone rang. It was Alison. She proceeded to tell me there is a neuromuscular clinic at the Children's Hospital of Philadelphia or CHOP. She explained about an online form I needed to complete in order to set up an appointment. My first prayer and it was answered in 15 minutes!

Then I got to thinking...I prayed with my pastor and I experienced the angel clouds. Then I prayed for direction and I was shown the way to go. Hard to explain away. My experiences did not end there. So when John & I filled out the form for CHOP the following day, we found that it needed to be faxed. Not having a fax machine we needed to make a trip to a copy center. John suggested I go just to get out of the house. Inside I was terrified I'd have another panic attack but agreed to go. Driving in the car I got stuck in traffic and of course a panic feeling started to come over me. I looked down and took a deep breath and on the radio I heard a line from the song playing; "faith is something you can't see." Then I looked up and on the rear window of the car in front of me was the simple word "faith." Okay this is getting weird. Then for some reason I started getting angry. I felt God answered my prayers so why can't he stop Duchenne from destroying my son's muscles. Why is this happening? So traffic began to move and a large truck merged in front of me. On the back of the truck was a single word I couldn't make out. KWITCHERBITCHIN! Translated into Quit Your Bitching! Oh so HE has a sense of humor too!

Things began to speed up from here because within 4 days we had our first appointment at CHOP. As we sat waiting for our new neurologist, Colin looked at me and asked me if he was sick. When I said no, he gave me a look that said why am I here. I told him we were getting his muscles checked out to see how strong they were. I'll never forget Colin asking me "Will I like this doctor?" He also realized how bad our first experience was. I really hoped we would like this new neurologist.

The first thing our new doctor did was look John and I right in the eye and ask how we were doing. I'm sure we looked awful since we were just given Colin's diagnosis 5 days earlier. He told us this is tough, the toughest thing imaginable, but if we can get ourselves together the better. The better we do, the better Colin will do. That message stuck with us. On the way home, when we asked Colin if he liked Dr. Finkel, he gave us a huge smile and shook his head YES!

The craziest thing was to learn that I could be a carrier for Duchenne Muscular Dystrophy. How could this be? I have 5 male cousins and an uncle and they have no muscle problems. Turns out it started with me. Colin and I share the same birthday, August 6th, and the same genetic deletion. Then on top of it my daughter, who was 1 at the time may also be a carrier. She will be tested when she is older. Our new doctor told us let's not worry about this right now. Having that knowledge won't change anything at this point. Will I never have grandchildren? How sad. Even now, a few people still ask me how did you NOT know about Colin's MD. Well for one thing he met all of his milestones within the range of what is considered typical. He was walking by 13 months which is not really typical for boys with Duchenne. The

ONLY glaring thing we noticed was by the age of 3 he could NOT jump. So instead of giving all that detail as a response, I simply say that God's timing is perfect. Had I known when Colin was a toddler that he had Duchenne and that I am a carrier, I would not have had any more children. I strongly believe that Colin was meant to have his sister, Sara. Her fierce independence encourages him be so also. She wrestles with him and plays silly games with him. She will pat him and tell him it is alright when his emotions get the best of him. She joins in with Colin's stretches and has asked for her own rocket boots but she requested "purple ones, please". Sara will mother Colin as only a little girl can. She will pat Colin and say "I'll take care of you." A lump forms in my throat when I think she could be a carrier and may never be a mother herself.

"The best way to make God laugh is tell Him your plans". I love that quote. There was a plan for John and I when we decided to get married. Never did I think that after John became a Tall Cedar* in the Masonic organization would our family have such an intimate experience with muscular dystrophy. One of the first steps in becoming a Mason is for a few brothers to visit the candidate and his family. I held 3 month old Colin in my arms explaining that the Tall Cedars commitment to supporting the Muscular Dystrophy Association was important to me. Colin has become the 2011 Goodwill Ambassador for the organization. We're all really proud of that. In fact when I look back just 6 years prior to Colin's diagnosis, I realize God's hand was guiding us towards the perfect house. John and I were interested in a beautiful house just down the road from where we currently live. One night the owner called me and asked for our final offer. A little voice in my head said "let it go." I did but couldn't understand why it wasn't to be. I was angry about that. Six years later we learned why a house with bedrooms on the second floor and a large set of steps up to the front porch wouldn't be for us.

In the end we built a comfortable ranch style home on a relatively flat piece of land.

My God moments showed me that even though I am not entirely in control of what happens in my life, I should not be afraid. Just trust and you will be shown the way. So back to that bittersweet gift. If not for Duchenne Muscular Dystrophy I would not have noticed these moments of pure love from dearly departed grandparents and a higher power. But if you think every day is easy just putting my trust in the Big Man, I assure you it is not. Just watching something as simple as Colin descending the bus steps can cause great joy, anger, sadness, and immense pain all at the same time. Colin slowly descends the steps when other boys jump off the last step. I never again will dismiss the little things in life because those little things are like giant steps for our sons. As I finish our story, I think so much of my young carefree daughter Sara. Will she feel as carefree as she gets older and comes to understand the cruelty of Duchenne? Or will she feel strengthened by it and develop a desire in her heart to see it end? I certainly hope the latter. It is possible for an ordinary everyday person like myself to rise up to the challenge and help give a voice to our sons and daughters. I will not be a victim but a force to be reckoned with.

*Cindy Studlack*

# Kevin, 9 Years Old

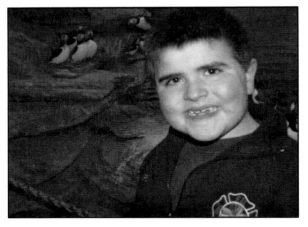

Kevin Peter Kearney is a funny, compassionate, lovable nine-year-old boy who physically, mentally, and emotionally drains me every day; and I wouldn't change a thing…except to have a cure for Duchenne Muscular Dystrophy (DMD).

Kevin was born on October 7, 2002. Big brother Brian was 5 ½ years old and big sister Shannon was 3 ½ years old. I will never forget the look on Brian's face when he first saw his baby brother. It was precious! We have a photo of Shannon holding Kevin and giving him the sweetest kiss! Everything was perfect; we had a healthy 9 pound 1 ounce baby boy. We took him home 2 days later. Kevin was a great baby except that he slept ALL DAY and was awake ALL NIGHT! I was exhausted! Eventually, his sleeping habits changed and he was sleeping better at night. We were tired but we were happy! We had three perfectly healthy children. Our lives were busy. The children were growing quickly.

When Kevin was three months of age we had a photographer come to our house to take a photo. The photographer propped him up on pillows. We tried to get Kevin to smile but he wouldn't because he was so miserable. It was extremely difficult for him to hold his head up. I thought to myself, why is Kevin having so much trouble? But I didn't worry too much about it. I knew children developed differently. Weeks went by and, according to the first year baby book, Kevin should have been rolling over, but he wasn't. In time he did roll over, but it was later than average. I still wasn't worried.

The next milestone was crawling. Kevin never crawled. He scooted. He sat on his rear end and used his arm to lift off the ground to cruise around the room. I read that some children just prefer scooting to crawling. Again, I wasn't too worried. Kevin turned one year old. He was developing a personality but he was nowhere near being able to walk. I finally began to worry. My husband, Peter, did as well. We took him for his yearly physical. The pediatrician agreed with our concerns and suggested we see a neurologist. The neurologist told us that Kevin should begin physical therapy and that we should come back for a follow-up visit in a few months. He began physical therapy and took a few steps at about 16 months of age. At 17 months, we went back to the neurologist. He wanted us to get a blood test just to "rules some things out". He did not seem overly concerned so we didn't rush to get the test done.

About three weeks later we went for the blood test. The next day the neurologist, not the nurse or the secretary, but the neurologist himself, called us. He wanted to speak with us in person as soon as possible. I knew it was bad. A doctor doesn't call you himself and want to speak with you immediately unless it is something bad. Still, I just thought he was going to tell us that Kevin had a vitamin deficiency. He had mentioned something about that during our first visit with him. He talked his "doctor talk' telling us that the CPK blood test results were very high and that could only mean MUSCULAR DYSTROPHY. I felt like someone had punched me in the stomach. That is the only way I can describe how I felt! I remember the doctor visibly having a hard time telling us this horrible news. I remember getting teary eyed. I remember Peter asking a few questions. I don't remember much else that happened in the office except that the doctor told us NOT to go online. He said it would be too overwhelming. I did not follow his advice. I went home and immediately googled the words: muscular dystrophy. I had to find out more information. The only thing I knew about muscular dystrophy was what I had learned from the Jerry Lewis Telethon that I used to watch every Labor Day weekend when I was a child. After reading online for a little while, I learned that there are many different forms of muscular dystrophy. We eventually learned that the form of muscular dystrophy that Kevin had was the most common form, Duchenne. Our lives have not been the same since that day in April of 2004. My heart began to break that day. It breaks a little more every day.

After we learned of Kevin's diagnosis, I was in a fog. It was like I was living a dream. I couldn't believe this was happening. I couldn't believe I had one of "Jerry's Kids". I still cannot believe my youngest son has this horrific disease. Some people would have buried their head in the sand, crawled into bed for weeks, or went into complete denial. Not me. I spent hours reading about DMD. I couldn't get enough information. All I wanted was to get Kevin the help he needed. The week before his second birthday a bus came to pick him up to take him to a special education pre-school where he received physical therapy, occupational therapy, and speech therapy. Many people have told me that they wouldn't have been able to send their two year old on a bus by himself. I was a little anxious, but I knew it would be the best thing for him. He had a big smile on his face as he waved good bye on that first day of school. But school was, and still is, not all smiles. Kevin has many difficulties in school physically, academically, and behaviorally. He has been in self-contained special education classes for all of his elementary school years. It has been so difficult for me, as a teacher, to see him dread school work so much. I have put so much of my energy into trying to make learning fun for him. Seeing him having so much difficulty in school makes my heart break a little more each day.

Watching Kevin struggle with every single thing he does has been so incredibly difficult. The other day he said to me, "Look how high I can jump Mommy!", and he had one foot one the ground and lifted the other a few inches off the floor. Inside my heart continued to break, but on the outside I said "That's really high Kevin!", with a big smile on my face. Last week he said to me, "Look how strong I am Mommy", as he carried in a bag of groceries containing a loaf a bread and a couple of other light items. Again, my heart broke a little more on the inside, but I said with a smile, "Yes, Kevin you are so strong!" I should win an Academy Award for my performances.

We are at the point in the disease where Kevin is having difficulty getting up from the floor. He calls for me to help him up and sometimes when I do he says, "Sorry to bother you Mommy." This disease is not fair. It is not fair that a little boy should have to apologize for needing help to get up off the ground. It is not fair that a little boy has never been able to jump with both feet. It is not fair that he has never been able to run or ride a two wheeler bike. It is not fair that when he goes to a birthday party he avoids the jumpy castle because he doesn't have the strength to stand as all the other kids are jumping. It is not fair to the rest of the family to have to watch the little boy struggle so much. The crack in my heart grows bigger.

Duchenne. It's a word I don't remember ever hearing before April of 2004. Now it's a word I can never get out of my head. Duchenne is on my mind every minute of every day....24/7. When I am reading a book or the newspaper, I am thinking about Duchenne. When I am watching TV or a movie, Duchenne is on my mind. When I am at work teaching first grade or listening to my principal during a faculty meeting, Duchenne is in my thoughts. Even though I am thinking about this disease constantly, I don't talk about it much because I don't want people to pity me and I don't want to be a downer. Sometimes I wish I could constantly talk about Duchenne to spread awareness. The world needs to know more about Duchenne. I wish I could tell everyone the reason why we need to find a cure for this terrible disease. I wish I could tell everyone how horrible it feels to know my son won't live long, how he probably won't go away to college, and he probably won't get married and have children. All the dreams I had for Kevin are demolished. We need to find a cure!

Words cannot describe how it feels to have a child with a fatal disease. I constantly feel badly that I am not able to give my two older children more attention. Brian and Shannon have to deal with so much because they have such a needy brother. My firefighter husband was strong enough to survive 9/11, but the pain of Duchenne is written all over his face. There are some days when I am so exhausted and I feel I can't handle this disease anymore. There are times when I think about the future and the care that Kevin will need and I wonder how I'll be able to handle it all. I can barely handle things now and I am in the "easy part" of this disease. There have been many times when I have completely lost it emotionally. I have gone into hysterics and cried myself to sleep. But I get up the next day and start all over again. I go to church every Sunday and pray every day for God to give me strength. I pray for the day when my heart will stop breaking. As time goes on, I get stronger and stronger. I know God won't give me more than I can handle and I put the negative, stressful thoughts, and the thoughts of the future, out of my mind. My motto is "Day By Day".

I have been able to make it through "Day By Day" because of the wonderful people in my life. First and foremost, my supportive husband and amazing children are always there for me. I wouldn't be able to survive without the help of my parents, Eileen and Jack McAdams and my mother-in-law, Dympna (sp?) Kearney (and my late father-in-law Peter Kearney). I am very lucky to have so many wonderful friends, especially my best friend, Bernadette Kowalchuk. My colleagues and friends at Richard P. Connor School have made me laugh on many days when all I wanted to do was cry. I am truly appreciative of the terrific people in my town of Orangetown, New York, and the surrounding communities who have been extremely supportive. You all are helping me mend my broken heart.

*Eileen Kearney*

# Nicholas, 9 Years Old

## Our Seal of Courage

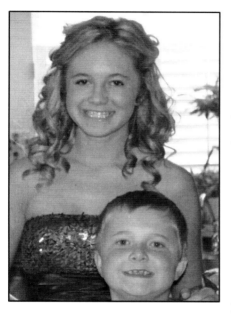

My name is Sherri Ritter. My son, Nicholas, was diagnosed with Duchenne in 2011 at eight years old. I always had a strong feeling that something wasn't quite right with the way he ran or got up from the floor. After repeated attempts at the pediatrician's office and orthopedic doctors, I felt assured that all was okay with Nicholas.

Let me go back about 28 years ago when my nephew, Joshua, was diagnosed with Duchenne. It was quite devastating that this beautiful young boy had such a horrible, cruel illness. I found that only we, as adults, were devastated. My nephew enjoyed life and is now 32 years old and in a nursing home because most doctors are uneducated about how to treat adults with MD. My nephew's spirit lives in us all, and when I have a bad day, I think of him, and it puts a smile on my face.

When Joshua was diagnosed, I was tested to determine if I was a carrier. The results were negative. Several years later, I was married and started a family. My first-born was a girl, Victoria. She was beautiful and flowing with life. A few years later, we decided to have another child. After repeated attempts that failed, we consulted a fertility specialist who decided a genetic test for DMD wasn't necessary due to the fact I had tested negative 25 years ago. After a few doses of Clomid, I was pregnant. Nicholas had a normal birth on May 23, 2003, his exact due date. Life was great. The doctors told me that Nicholas was fine and that any concerns I had were unwarranted.

On February 12, 2011, Nicholas was at his cousin's birthday party and on his feet all day. My niece called and said something was wrong with Nicholas. I had to carry him out of the party, but I wasn't overly concerned. I gave him some Motrin, but over the course of the next few days, I realized how large his calves were. People always said that he had football-player calves, and I noticed more of a Gower's Movement when he was getting off the floor. I immediately took him to the doctors, who ordered blood work stat, meaning right away. That evening changed my life forever. The doctor called us and said that Nicholas had a CPK level over 35,000. My heart sank because, after dealing with my nephew, I knew exactly what that meant. Over the next few days, I was panicked. I asked the doctor to repeat the test. The CPK level was then at 27,000. I then consulted a friend of mine, Dr. Oska, and said, "I don't believe this. I tested negative years ago. Please test for other conditions." So I had Nicholas tested for every other possible disorder involving CPK abnormalities, and they all came back negative.

At this point, I made an appointment to meet with an MDA Specialist whom I've known because of my nephew. I recall Maggie the Coordinator remembering me with tears in her eyes. She reassured me that they were so close to a cure that we could battle this disease. The DNA test was ordered. This was the longest four weeks I had to wait in my life. The doctor called my husband's cell phone because I was at my daughter's hockey party. When I saw his face, I knew immediately Nicholas had MD. I wanted more information. I came home, scoured the computer, and became a Do It Yourself scientist overnight. I tore apart the exons and chromosomes and really understood the duplication of Exons 13-21, and thought I had saved the world. All they had to do was take out the extras, right?

This activity continued for weeks. I was short with the kids and struggled at work and with my personal life. Duchenne consumed me. Google did not have enough information. I had already gone through every search engine. At one point, I had three appointments set up at the various Muscular Dystrophy Association locations in the Detroit Metro Area. I knew how to do this from dealing with my nephew. The biopsy was scheduled, but that was two months away. This was unacceptable to me, so I called and called until I found a surgeon to perform the biopsy. Finally, the madness slowed down when I came in contact with a parent in my area from the PPMD website. After conversing with Jen, I realized, after all, that there were other "scientists" out there like me, and our boys were very similar. I told her how frustrated I was with having to tell each and every doctor the entire story. It was as if they never talked to each other. I wanted a team to work for my son, and Detroit does not offer this. She told me about Cincinnati Children's Hospital. I researched the team and Dr. Wong. I then decided to take a step back and make the appointment. In the meantime, Nicholas' biopsy results came back— another stab in the gut. He had zero dystrophin. According to the pathologist, this was not good. It meant he had a severe case of DMD. I turned into a "pathologist," then, and felt better when I realized that the test did not include the western blot staining.

I prayed and prayed and asked for God's help to have the patience to wait for my Cincinnati appointment. It worked. Before I knew it, our appointment was there. I wanted to make this a memorable event, so I took along Nick's good friend, Nolan, and my old friend from high school, Lisa. I was highly impressed at the heart-warming feeling we received when we went to the hospital. Nolan kept Nick's spirits up by making jokes, telling Nick everything was going to be fine, and then showing him how to take funny pictures of all the doctors with the DS and the IPod Touch. This is what Nick's life is about, not the tests, not the disease, but living life to the fullest. Now Nolan and Nick call each other Bros and are already planning what they are going to do at the next visit to Cincinnati. Beware, staff at Cincinnati. You may end up on You Tube.

Then the muscle MRI test was done. Dr. Wong came running in with the results and said Nick's results showed a mild form of Duchenne. Nicholas was a candidate for Prednisone therapy. My nephew had no options when he was diagnosed and, for this, I was grateful that we had some, even though very few, options.

As we continue through this journey fighting day after day against this disease, not once have I said I was going to give up. A blow like this to your family causes a lot of strain and in the midst of all this, steroids cause excessive rage that cannot be controlled. You either accept my child for who he is and love him, or you're not part of our circle. My husband is one of those who cannot handle these rages, and we have decided to separate amicably. My dream was to have a supporting partner in sharing this fight, but the passion just is not there, although he loves his son dearly and would do anything for him. Some of us are just more passionate about life. As we move forward, treating Nicholas like a normal child is difficult. It takes every ounce of energy that I have not to have him by my side 24/7.

A very good friend of mine is a Harley lover, and because of the history of my nephew, I knew that Harley was one of the biggest promoters to raise money for muscular dystrophy. I instantly had an idea and proposed it as a partnered investment and as an effort to raise awareness in our community for muscular dystrophy and autism. My friend's son, Michael, is severely autistic. Having any type of special needs child is difficult. It irritates me the way people stare and do not teach their children that all of these kids are God's children, as well. Whenever I took my nephew to public places, I would make a point to inform people exactly what they were looking at. This may have been a bit aggressive, but anyone who knows me realizes that this is my normal way of being. I even installed a horn on his electric wheelchair, just for the fun of it!

Our project consists of rebuilding and restoring a 1958 Harley. Mike's boys, Nolan, Nathan, Michael and my son, Nicholas, were equipped with tool boxes and Harley gear because they are now part of the crew. Not only is this a wonderful experience for the boys, but it has a very meaningful purpose for the both of us. I am taking a proposal to our local Harley dealership and promoting a bike run in our county to raise awareness for both causes. My next project is a dinner/dance fundraiser to raise money for the MD Association and for Nicholas' medical trust fund, to be tapped when and if we need to make modifications to our house.

I am very hopeful that all of these trial studies and research groups are successful for all of our boys. It just breaks my heart to hear about so many of these boys that I know who have passed away. Nicholas is a very outgoing, energetic child, and I do not want to ever hold him back from achieving any of his goals. Just remember, your child is still your child, and leading a normal life and being grateful are very important in living with this disease. Just like anything in life, if it's meant to happen, it will happen. Just keep fighting for what you want.

On an ending note, remember, we are our child's advocate. My goal is to advocate for these boys with Duchenne, whether they are an adult or child. We are their only hope. Do not take NO for an answer and keep pushing forward. God does not give us any more than we can handle. Use your resources wisely and get a good circle of FRIENDS for support. I truly believe that everything happens for a reason. Maybe God is humbling us all and telling us to slow down and look at life through the beauty, not through the glass window.

Finally— Enjoy Life, Live Simply, Have Fun, and Love a Lot and cherish that circle of friends that matters in your present life. And most of all, remember that God is with you. Amen

*Sherri Ritter*

## Nathan, 10 Years Old

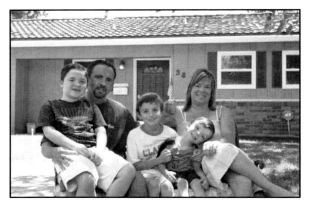

Much of what I know about being a father, I learned from my dad. I have admired him for as long as I can remember. He was a scholarship athlete in college and a graduate of Stanford University who majored in engineering. My dad also fulfilled his military obligation as a reservist in the army as a Green Beret, and was able to feed, clothe, and offer the opportunity of a college education to each of his seven children as result of his diligence and strong work ethic as a construction executive. When we were growing up, my brothers, sisters, and I lived by a simple code: if you're going to get in trouble, find Mom; if you're already really in trouble, get Dad. There was nothing he could not fix. To me, he has always been the quintessential father figure—the provider and protector—the embodiment of strength.

While I have known that he and I have vastly different talents and abilities, I always imagined that my role as a father would follow a similar path to his when it became time to start a family of my own. I hoped that my family would always know the safety and security I felt as a child. My plan seemed to be on track when my first child Matthew was born. I imagined coaching my children in sports, taking them on camping trips, even working in the yard together. My wife Wendy gave birth to my second son Nathan a short time later and everything seemed to be working according to plan until Nathan broke his femur at age two. We were scared, but the doctors assured us that he would be okay. We were able to see his determination for the first time when, despite a cast that covered his entire leg and spanned most of his chest, Nathan taught himself to walk again within a week's time. While he mended quickly, concern nagged at both of us.

He never seemed to have the bounce in his step that other boys his age had. In the beginning, we assumed that he was still recovering from his injury. Wendy and I talked about the fall, and that there was something about the way he fell that seemed unnatural. Something was not right. Why would a leg injury make it difficult for him to stand up from the floor? Eventually, maternal instincts prevailed and Wendy insisted on further evaluation. We had no idea about the odyssey we were about to begin.

Our pediatrician evaluated Nathan and said she suspected he might have muscular dystrophy. That afternoon, I searched the Internet and it took me to the MDA website where I narrowed my results to Becker and Duchenne because of his young age (he was 5 at the time.). I read the descriptions repeatedly. I remember thinking, "As long as it's not Duchenne, we'll be fine; we can handle Becker, but not the other one." Finally, the pediatric neurologist confirmed the worst possibility—Duchenne. Adding to the confusion, we found out a week later that Wendy was pregnant.

The possibility that another of our sons would be born with a disease that we did not understand overshadowed our joyous news. With each appointment, our physicians would as ask if Wendy wanted to terminate her pregnancy. There was no way we could make that decision, but we were lost and did not know what to do. From the time Nathan was diagnosed until his baby brother Josh was born, Nathan spent every night nestled between us in our bed. All we could think to do was to hold him tight. Thankfully, Josh does not have muscular dystrophy.

Six years have passed since the diagnosis, and we have experienced a myriad of emotions. Initially, the steroids bolstered Nathan's strength and he was able to keep up with his peers. Life appeared normal for a while, but we began to see changes. As the effects of Nathan's disease have become more apparent, reality has set in. In the matter of a few months, he stopped being able to walk independently. We often explain that he walked into third grade and rolled out of it. The wheelchair pulled us from denial and made us realize that we needed to take a more immediate and active role in our son's life.

We now operate with a much greater sense of urgency. One lesson we have learned from Duchenne is that time is precious. Like other parents and caregivers of Duchenne children, when I lift and move him, I constantly steal opportunities to hug him. I have never put him to bed at night without squeezing him a little extra, "because I can." Wendy, in particular, has become a champion for our son. Thanks to her efforts, we are working with canine companions to match Nathan with a dog to provide him with assistance. She also reached out to Make-a-Wish so that Nathan can fully participate in his once-in-a-lifetime experience. I try to follow her lead as she makes every effort to celebrate life as much as possible with Nathan.

My role as a father has been redefined. Serving as my family's provider and protector as I had originally envisioned is a dream that I will never realize. I, unlike my dad, have to rely on others for help. For me, like parents of all disabled children, it is an extremely helpless feeling to see the fear in my son's eyes and know I am unable to fix it or "make it better." We are not able to engage in many of the same activities as other fathers and sons. I not only worry about excluding Nathan when I play with his brothers, but I also feel like they are being robbed of experiences. I combat this feeling, however, by simply resolving myself to do what I can, when I can, however I can. And while it never seems sufficient, and it typically feels like none of the boys is happy, this is when I feel like every other parent—whether their children are healthy or not. Nothing is, or ever will be, good enough for our children.

Family and friends have been an amazing source of support for our family when we have needed it most. Wendy's parents have been amazing throughout Nathan's life. Little did they know that they *retired* to work as hard as they do as the boys' primary caretakers while we are working. We have often said that one of the few positives that come from the disease is realizing how many people truly care for us.

Although we feel that Duchenne is a cruel disease, we know that we are extremely lucky to have been given an opportunity to learn the meaning of love in a way that was formerly beyond our comprehension. In the coming years, Wendy, Matthew, Nathan, Josh, and I look forward to making memories and smiles that will last a lifetime. We hope to draw from Nathan's dogged determination and enduring strength of spirit. Muscular Dystrophy has taught us the value of time, and we are committed to maximizing every opportunity we have with each other. While others may squabble and squander their time as a family, we cannot waste our precious time together. We do not yet understand why we were chosen for this path, but we trust that there is a reason and that one day it will become self-evident. In the meantime, we will try to relish and fight for every moment together, remaining hopeful that a greater future than we can yet imagine awaits us.

"That which we are, we are; One equal temper of heroic hearts, Made weak by time and fate, but strong in will to strive, to seek, to find, and not to yield."
**~Ulysses, Alfred Lord Tennyson**

*Paul St. Geme*

# James, 10 and Jacob 7 Years Old

*O give thanks unto the LORD; for He is good: because*
*His mercy endures forever. ~Psalm 118*

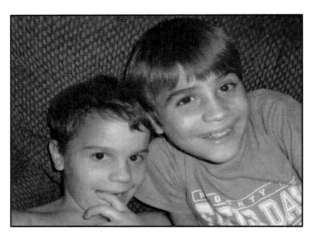

Thank you so much for reading our story! I am a blessed and deeply loved wife and mother of seven beautiful children, four daughters and three sons. On May 5, 2010, our oldest son, James, who had just turned nine, was diagnosed with Duchenne Muscular Dystrophy. Our middle son, Jacob, who also has autism, was diagnosed several months later. Our youngest son, Joshua, was spared the disease.

We thank God for our children every day and trust that His plans are equally good for each of them. Our sweet children have been instrumental in minimizing the impact of this disease on our family. I hope getting to know our family will encourage you to join the fight to End Duchenne!

*"Then the **dove** came to him in the evening, and behold, a freshly plucked olive leaf was in her mouth; and Noah knew that the waters had receded from the earth." ~Genesis 8:11*

Our oldest child, Dove, our beautiful "brown-eyed girl," has maturity beyond her years. Indeed, there are very few girls her age that could care for six younger children, yet she handles it with ease. Dove has such a nurturing spirit and at the same time has an incredible ability to take control of any situation. She is such an encouragement to all of her siblings, helps to provide round-the-clock care to her brother Jacob and is committed to James' critical stretching regimen. As I watch Dove with her siblings each day, I see her become more amazingly beautiful inside and out!

*"But those who hope in the LORD will renew their strength. They will soar on wings like eagles; they will run and not grow weary, they will walk and not be faint." ~Isaiah 40:31*

Our second-oldest daughter, Sarai Hope, is such a sweet and loving young lady. She takes over much of the motherly role; each morning she welcomes the younger children with big hugs and reads stories to them at night. The combination of her dramatic personality along with her interests makes her an ideal companion for Jacob. It is amazing how long she can maintain his attention by demonstrating to him how to make a key-lime pie or teaching him a computer game. Sarai loves to pet Jacob's hair and entertains him with silly faces or dances with him to his favorite music.

*"My grace is sufficient for you, for my power is made perfect in weakness. Therefore I will boast all the more gladly about my weaknesses, so that Christ's power may rest on me. That is why, for Christ's sake, I delight in weaknesses, in insults, in hardships, in persecutions, in difficulties. For when I am weak, then I am strong." ~2Cor 12:9-10*

Tabitha Grace is our middle child, everyone's best friend, always on your side no matter whose side you're on. She is a very talented, silly and pretty little girl. Tabitha is sandwiched in between James and Jacob, twenty months on each side, and has special relationships with both of them. She has taken a caretaking role with Jacob, whom she calls her *buddy*. She leads him to his class and takes over at home when her older sisters are unavailable. She also is the biggest helper when Jacob has lessons at home, often taking notes for his teacher. Tabitha and James are the best of friends, and I can't imagine either one without the other.

*"The LORD gave this command to Joshua son of Nun: "Be strong and courageous, for you will bring the Israelites into the land I promised them on oath, and I myself will be with you." ~Deuteronomy 31:23*

Our youngest son, Joshua, is very much a typical little boy, active and strong. He can turn anything into a sword and is quite nimble when it comes to a mock sword fight. We often hear wild sounds coming from the boys' room and find Joshua and James rolling on the floor play-fighting. Thankfully, Joshua is also very intuitive and considerate. He recognizes when James has had enough activity and will end the fight or let big brother win. He is so tender-hearted and usually the first to come to the rescue. He realized at a very young age that Jacob was special and needed his help. It warms my heart when I find Joshua comforting Jacob or referring to James as his "best brother".

*"The women said to Naomi: "Praise be to the LORD, who this day has not left you without a kinsman-redeemer." ~Ruth 4:13-17*

Our baby girl, Naomi Joy, was born nearly two years before we got the news of the boys' illness. Our little blond blue-eyed beauty is the cutest thing in the world, truly a joy! Like most three-year-old girls, Naomi is such a busy body, absorbing every bit of information. Although she wants to become a "big girl," she's obviously perfectly content being the baby of the family. James simply adores her and she can charm him into anything!

*"Blessed are those whose help is the God of Jacob, whose hope is in the LORD their God." ~Psalm 146:5*

Our beautiful middle son, Jacob, was an incredibly easy-going baby, quiet, yet very friendly. He continues to be a very happy little boy, content with so many people loving and taking care of him. Jacob still doesn't speak, but he is clearly very bright and understands just about everything spoken to him. He is strong and likes to climb, often getting in trouble when he does. He loves water, sand, music and lots of hugs!

*"Consider it pure joy, my brothers and sisters, whenever you face trials of many kinds, because you know that the testing of your faith produces perseverance. Let perseverance finish its work so that you may be mature and complete, not lacking anything." ~James 1:2-4*

James is such a pleasant young man, determined to please. He is respectful and cooperative, kind and considerate, handsome and bright. He also is an amazing help with his younger brothers and sisters. I find it so amazing that James had this disease that was wearing his muscles down for nine years before it was discovered. To this day, he has not let it wear him down and he continues to be an active boy. He loves to ride his bike, jump on the trampoline, surf the waves, and play ball. He also enjoys swimming, dancing, singing, playing the drums and harmonica as well as being an accomplished artist and inventor.

He is incredibly optimistic, always keeping in mind the promises of God. Recently, my husband read Zechariah 8:5 to the children, *"And the streets of the city shall be full of boys and girls playing in the streets thereof."* James recognized the message that heaven will be fun and safe, no dangers and no more sorrow and, as he commented, "There will be no more diseases!"

*"May your God, whom you serve continually, rescue you!" "For he is the living God and he endures forever; his kingdom will not be destroyed, his dominion will never end.*

*He rescues and he saves; he performs signs and wonders in the heavens and on the earth." ~Daniel 6:16, 26-27*

I am so very thankful for my wonderful husband, Jimmy, who is my support, my encouragement, my love. Soon after the diagnosis, Jimmy had the urge to spend time with his oldest son and took him on a summer road trip. It was a memorable time for all of us, as we were invited to join them at times. Jimmy is indeed an adventurous and entertaining daddy, but he is also a fighter and prayer warrior. Like the patriarch Jacob, Jimmy continues to wrestle with God to receive the blessing for his sons and, like the Psalmist David, prays for them without ceasing.

Indeed, Jimmy is a constant reminder of the promises of God. He is like Daniel, remaining faithful regardless of the outcome, and the Apostle Paul, a constant reminder that His grace is sufficient. Most notably he wholeheartedly believes in Jesus' words when He proclaimed that with faith, and by the power of God, we can move mountains. He truly is the best husband and father, and I couldn't imagine going through this journey without him.

*"So Jesus answered and said to them, "Assuredly, I say to you, if you have faith and do not doubt, if you say to this mountain, 'Be removed and be cast into the sea,' it will be done. And whatever things you ask in prayer, believing, you will receive." ~Matt21:21-22*

We have many challenges ahead, but we are trusting in the Lord and His perfect goodness, purpose and mercy. We certainly will no longer take for granted a moment of the time we have with all of our children. We have been humbled by so many special people who have offered us their help, guidance and prayers. Most of all we are so thankful to the Lord for the grace He has shown in the lives of James and Jacob and the immense blessing they are to our family.

*"Rejoice evermore. Pray without ceasing. In everything give thanks: for this is the will of God in Christ Jesus concerning you." ~ Thessalonians 5:16-18*

*Stacy Daniels*

## *The Race: By Sarai, sister of James and Jacob (age 12)*

It came from the start, without us knowing, that broke our hearts, and their bodies kept on slowing.

Two boys with hearts as long as a pole, just keep on racing, and that is their goal.

Not stopping without a prayer and never looking back, where no one is there, but always looking up, ready to be packed.

When they cross the finish line, they will be greeted by a bigger family, and certainly will shine, that's where they will be, thankfully.

And then they will walk in peacefulness and joy and their hearts never will be destroyed.

### My Brothers James and Jacob: By Tabitha (age 8)

James and Jacob are my brothers. They are very nice and I love playing with them. James and I are pals. We always play with each other. Even though James is older than I, I still take care of him, but he gets mad at me when I do. When I tell Jacob not to go somewhere, he might scream, but he doesn't mean to be bad. Sometimes people in our school make fun of them and I don't like it. Jacob doesn't talk, but he's smart, so don't laugh at him. James is slow, but you shouldn't make fun of him and call him a slow poke because that is mean. If you see James or Jacob fall, then you should ask, "Are you ok?" Then help them up. I love my brothers and you should, too!

# Kyle, 11 Years Old

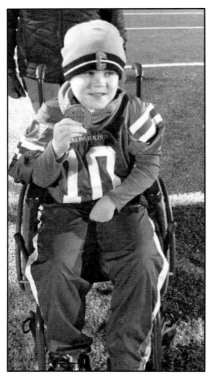

### Three Distinct Days

There are momentous days in each of our lives. I want to share three of those days that have shaped our family.

### Sept 2, 2000

The anticipation was palpable. This was our first child and the first grandchild on both sides of the family. We knew he was going to be a boy. Jill had checked into the hospital on Friday morning. Finally, in the early evening on Saturday, she had a c-section to bring Kyle into this world. I remember the first time I saw him. He was being held by the nurse, and he was scrunched up with his eyes closed. He was perfect. It was both exciting and tiring and was the beginning of an adventure. We were in our mid-twenties, and we were ready for this new stage of life with kids.

This was just the beginning. The possibilities were endless. Sports had played such a huge role in my life, and I was positive that they would play an integral role in Kyle's life, also. The first thing we did as father and son was watch a football game. I remember it well. It was opening day of the season. It was the Bears against the Vikings. Cade McNown had one of his best days as a pro. The Bears won and life was good.

At about six months, we knew something wasn't right. Kyle was a great baby, but he wasn't functioning as a "normal" baby. He wasn't rolling over; he wasn't sitting up on his own. Throughout the next couple of years we kept hearing the word "delay." Kyle was just delayed, it wasn't anything to worry about, with physical therapy he would catch up. No one seemed overly worried, so we were patient. When he was two-and-a-half, we decided to take him to Riley's Children Hospital in Indianapolis. During that visit we had a blood test with various other tests done. It would be about a week before we would receive the results.

## A Wednesday in February of 2003

It was a typical morning. I had left for work around 8:30 and had been at my desk for about half an hour when the secretary told me Jill was on the phone. Jill calmly and softly told me the blood test had come back, and the doctors believed Kyle had muscular dystrophy. The first question was, "What does this mean?" Jill said something to the effect that she didn't have any idea. My head was spinning, and immediately I did an Internet search of muscular dystrophy. It didn't take long for my world to crash around me. As I sat in my office at the church where I worked, I sobbed. I was sitting in a place where people find hope, peace, and comfort, but I was feeling despair, hopelessness, and anxiety.

We didn't initially know what type of muscular dystrophy Kyle would have. There was hope in the initial stages that he would have something other than Duchenne. We quickly learned that Duchenne was the most common form of MD, and it was likely that Kyle had this. I didn't know all the implications but I did know that this would change our lives.

There were good days and bad for the next few years. I didn't know how to respond or react. I am not sure I still know how. There was a loss: Kyle wouldn't be the person I thought he would be. There was so much gut-wrenching pain in that. Each time I was hit by the thought of things we wouldn't experience together, I would undergo a new wave of emotion.

## Today:

There is a huge difference between existing and living. For much of the last eight years, our family was breathing and existing. But we weren't living.

I was disengaged most of the time, trying to escape reality by being overly involved in work, projects, and leisure enjoyments. There were many titles and roles I was comfortable with, but father of a special needs child was not one of them. I didn't have a road map for what I was supposed to do or how I was to act.

Then the summer of 2011 came. There were two catalytic moments that changed our (specifically my) life and our relationship to Duchenne. The first was going to a family camp put on for special needs families by Joni and Friend's ministry. For three years, our church had tried to talk our family into going. I had dragged my feet and had not wanted to do it. I was very uncomfortable with the thought of going to a place where I would have to face reality for a week. I was voted down four to one in our family vote for attending the camp. It was that week that began the reengagement for me. Seeing and meeting other fathers who had dealt with the same moments I had was therapeutic. We laughed, cried, and bonded so quickly over our common crisis in life. Seeing these examples was what I needed.

The other moment that changed our perspective was when we received a call from a local foot doctor who asked if he could have Kyle do a sprint triathlon with him. We (I) had focused so long on Kyle's limitations that we had not allowed him to live life. The triathlon opened up possibilities that we never had thought of before. After the triathlon, Kyle began asking to do activities he had never known before, like sky diving Our conversations began to center on how Kyle could do something, rather than lamenting why he couldn't. Today is such an important day in Kyle's life, because we can't wait to see what he can do. We can't wish that he didn't have this disease; we can't feel sorry for ourselves or for Kyle.

*Matthew 6:34- "So don't worry about tomorrow, for tomorrow will bring its own worries.*
*Today's trouble is enough for today."*

We can't wake up every morning scared of the future. We can't dwell on all the horrific moments, but rather can have peace in the moments of today. Today is a great day because we have the privilege and opportunity to spend it with Kyle. Each day brings laughs, tears and moments that will never be forgotten.

I have missed out on moments in Kyle's life due to my fear and trepidation about his future. No, his life didn't turn out the way I expected, but no child's does. I believe that Kyle is fearfully and wonderfully made by a Creator who knows and loves him. Jill and I have been entrusted with Kyle's life, and as difficult as it is, we have made the choice that we are going to live one day at a time and not allow Duchenne to have the last word in our life. Yes, it is a reality, but it is not going to steal our joy or our peace or break up our family. Kyle will have a great day today. And that is what we are going to focus on.

*Ben Polhemus*

## Carlie, 11 Years Old

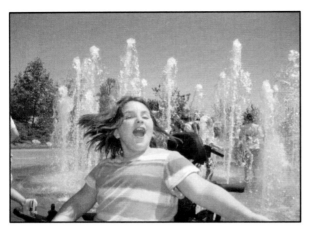

Carlie is my baby; my "Little Mary Sunshine". I was 38 when she was born, and she was tiny, beautiful, and perfect. She rolled over, crawled, and sat up just like her brothers and sister did. She stood up by 10 months, and walked not long after that. Carlie was doing everything when and how she was supposed to. As she got older, she would trip over "air" and had problems walking quickly. We just thought her short little legs just couldn't keep up. Then she started pre-school and we were told her gross and fine motor skills weren't where they should be, which led to a doctor visit. Dr. Annie checked her out; Carlie did everything she was asked to do: hop on one foot, step up onto a stool and off, jump up and down and more. Everything looked good, or so we thought. She was 3 years old.

In kindergarten they had more gross and fine motor concerns. Because of her young age, she was in kindergarten for 2 years. During this time she began having problems doing things like climbing the big step onto the bus. I had to help by "boosting" her up onto the top step. She also started having more problems doing ordinary things like climbing the front steps at home. She was also very unsteady on the playground at school, coming home with a huge goose egg because someone "tagged" her and caused her to fall and hit the sidewalk during recess. When we went to the store she would lag behind; her feet seemed to always slap the ground when she walked.

During first grade she began having very painful muscle cramps in her calves. She would cry because they hurt so badly. She would want to ride in the cart when we went to the grocery store because her legs would hurt and she would say she was tired. I just thought she wanted to ride in the cart, she was little and her legs were short. I thought she'd grow out of it in time…Once again we were referred to our family practitioner to evaluate the situation. He referred us to a pediatrician in his office. Carlie was 7 years old at the time. She never rode a bicycle, ever. She never got to play sports like basketball, or soccer, or any other game that involved running. When she did run and play, she would fall down on both knees. And every time, Carlie would pop right back up, "I'm OK!" she would say, usually with a smile on her face. She always had a smile on her face and lived up to my nickname for her *Little Mary Sunshine, my Angel Baby*. The pediatrician checked Carlie out and had her do all the things she'd been asked to do before. In the end we were told they weren't sure. The doctor said, "Usually after examining a child I can pretty well tell, but, with her, I just don't know."

Lab work was done before we left the office and we were told we would get a call with the results. It was the longest wait of my life. We received the call back and it was all I could do to maintain my composure, Carlie's CPK levels were in the 4,000's which was not good. The pediatrician referred us to Washington University Children's Hospital in St. Louis.

Carlie had an exam with Dr. Neal at the M.D. clinic there, and an appointment was made for a muscle biopsy. She was cast for leg braces but we just didn't know exactly what was going on.

The muscle biopsy went well and we waited for more results. We received a phone call just 2 weeks before Carlie's 8th birthday with a diagnosis of Limb-Girdle Muscular Dystrophy. It was June of 2008.

Somehow my older children and I just didn't think the diagnosis was accurate. We researched on-line and in books and we came to the conclusion that Carlie had Duchenne Muscular Dystrophy (DMD). We had seen commercials on television and Carlie had exactly the same symptoms as the boys we saw. Some of the symptoms were similar to Limb-Girdle, but it looked more like DMD than anything else. We went back to St. Louis for Carlie's 6-month check-up and the doctor looked at me and asked, "Are you familiar with Duchenne?" "Yes I am" was my reply as I thought "probably more than you are."

I felt like throwing up. I knew our lives were changed forever. How could I tell my sweet, precious, little girl that she was going to lose the ability to walk? And much more than that, how could our family come to terms with the fact we could possibly loose our baby...my baby, their baby sister?

I cried for 2 weeks after we got home. I was numb at the thought of what this all meant for our family, for Carlie. My sweet little Angel Baby....How could this be? What had I done for her to be burdened with this terrible disease? What were we going to do? My children are the best; my sons endured their father's battle with cancer and at 7 and 9, they lost their Daddy. Now they are faced with losing their baby sister who doesn't really understand what's happening. She knows the possibilities, but how real can they be to a 13-year old girl with so much to live for?

So we go on and we make the best of a rotten situation. We moved to a new place not far from where we were, so that Carlie could attend a better school district. Her school has done everything possible for her. When she started school in the '08-'09 school year, she could walk. By the summer of 2010 she was in a wheelchair full time. She could help hold herself up to assist with dressing and transferring, but within 6 months she lost those abilities too. At school they got a lift to assist with bathroom breaks as Carlie couldn't stand anymore.

What do you say to a child who has to spend all of her time sitting and watching the other kids play? When she looks at me and says "Mom, I wish I could walk." my heart breaks. Why can't I take this away from her? Why can't it be me? In 2 short years she went from walking to being in a chair full time. She went from being a happy, smiling little girl without a care in the world, to being a little girl with the weight of the world on her shoulders.

We try to stay positive; some days are better than others. We struggle with things like getting into the bathroom and tub on a daily basis. It's amazing how much a person takes for granted, when you can't do simple things like take a shower independently. If nothing else, this experience has helped us to have a better appreciation of the things we do have. And we try to appreciate each other more too. Our family was very close before Carlie's diagnosis, but I think we are even closer now. And I think we are more aware of others around us who are in need too. Our faith in God, and our love for one other is what keeps us strong.

*Kelly Frangella*

# Adam, 11 Years Old

## Defeat Is Not an Option
### By Laura Villeneuve (Adam's Sister)

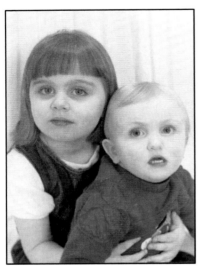

Let me just say right off the bat that I don't want your sympathy. My brother, Adam, is eleven (He turned 11 on 11/11/11) years old and has Duchenne Muscular Dystrophy (DMD). My name is Laura. I'm thirteen years old, and eight years ago, my life, along with the rest of my family's lives, changed forever.

Adam was four years old when he was diagnosed with DMD. I was only six, and I don't remember much of what happened back then. All I know is that my parents were devastated and scared. I don't remember feeling scared, just confused. The first memory I have of saying or knowing anything about DMD was when I was nine and shared a news article about DMD to my fourth grade class. I understood everything the article was saying, but no one, not even my teacher, knew anything. I didn't know how that could be, but as I explained DMD, I felt warm, as if sitting by a fire. That feeling I had has stayed with me all my life, and I still love that feeling. As I look back on it now, I believe it was obvious that I was feeling that way because I was doing a good deed.

Fourth grade was one of the best years of my life, and it changed me. It was during this time that I became inspired to help my brother and others with DMD. I have worked at multiple MDA events and am an advocate for raising money for Adam and others like him, including the annual MDA walk. It's my little way of helping that makes a big difference. In a way, I'm glad that I am part of a family that lives with DMD, because now I can contribute to finding a cure to save other people's lives and that warm feeling never goes away.

A few months ago, I was on the school bus with some of my peers, and we were talking about disabled kids. The others were saying how it would be nearly impossible for a person to live a disabled life, and I greatly disagreed. I told them that my brother lives a disabled life and he is doing very well. Everyone turned to look at me, minor shock on their faces by what I said, and I was a little surprised that they had known me for so long and didn't know about Adam. I told them Adam's story, and one girl said she was sorry, but I waved her off. She had nothing to be sorry for. It wasn't her fault Adam has DMD, and I was sick and tired of sympathy and apologies. I don't need those things. The only thing I need is doctors and researchers to do their jobs and find a cure for DMD.

I told Adam's story again a few days later. I was in advisory, and my teacher asked each of us to write down something that no one knew about us. I wrote down Adam's story, and I was given the opportunity to explain DMD again, but this time I was pretty certain that, at this age, most kids would be able to understand the story better and would listen in a different way than when they were nine.. A few of the people there had known me for years, and had heard Adam's story already, but others reacted the same way as they did four years ago. This didn't bug me as much, but I was still a little surprised that I had known these people for such a long time and they still didn't understand. DMD is a big part of my life, so I thought after six years they would have at least retained some of the knowledge from the other times I have talked about Adam.

I wish I could explain DMD to my entire school, but I couldn't do it with my siblings there. All three of my younger siblings are in elementary school and live with DMD as well, and I couldn't tell the story of our family on my own. Other times that I have talked about Adam and people's expressions have gone from curious to sympathetic. This drives me insane. Sympathy won't save Adam's life, so I don't need it. It brings me the opposite of comfort. People sometimes become extra careful because they are afraid that I am so upset about Adam that anything they say will make me start bawling. That is not the case at all. I have learned to live with a disabled brother.

DMD has taken an emotional toll on my life, and I have mixed feelings about it. Most days I forget about it entirely, but other times I wish I was in a different family. There was one instance a few years ago when Adam had gone into a classroom full of kids my age and they all commented to me later that they "couldn't believe how cute he was". For about a week I was only the girl with the cute little brother. This really upset me because I knew that people couldn't come to know me better if all they saw was Adam.

My life has also changed physically because of DMD. Our original house was not fit for a disabled person, much less a disabled young child. My parents decided to solve this problem by donating our house to the fire department. In 2008, the fire department burned down our house. My dad has built our new house to his specifications, meaning that it has elements that can be used by a handicapped person. This includes an elevator, a roll-in shower, and a wheelchair ramp.

Everyone is different and everyone has flaws, and Adam's is DMD. It is a big part of his life, but he is also loving, caring, respectful, funny, and sarcastic. I do worry about him though. He's in fifth grade now and from what I remember from my fifth grade year, my peers weren't that accepting of someone being different, and things that happen in fifth grade change people. The kids who bully Adam in fifth grade will continue to bully him all throughout junior high. I would hate to see Adam come home upset because people were teasing him. If he does, I think I'll need to have a talk with these kids. No one makes fun of my brother. I don't care how little you know, you should be smart enough to know that Adam is different, and he can't change.

Duchenne Muscular Dystrophy has changed my point of view on life. You only live once, and you shouldn't have to worry about a chronic disease. Adam doesn't need that. No one needs that. I can try my hardest to work toward a brighter future for Adam, but that's all I can do. I will work for him though, even if it means going to the extreme. If I was given the option to die and have all DMD patients be cured, or live and have only my brother saved, I would choose to die, because it wouldn't be right to see other families suffer and feel the guilt of only saving my brother. I would give my life to save every DMD patient, not only Adam. Defeat is not an option if someone's life is on the line, and I would rather die than surrender to Duchenne Muscular Dystrophy. I don't like thinking about what could happen if his disease becomes worse. Adam takes steroids every day to keep his muscle strength, and he has yet to be forced into a wheelchair. I think about him every day, and what could happen as he becomes older. One day my mom told me that Adam had had trouble falling asleep, and she told me it was because he was scared of the future. Kids with DMD have an increased chance of dying young, as early as the age of seventeen. Adam was scared that this was his fate. When I heard this, I wished instantly that the disease was gone and had never come near Adam or our family. I still wish for that, but since the disease is affecting Adam, the only thing I can do is try my hardest to raise money for him and pray that doctors and researchers find a cure before it's too late and the world loses another extraordinary little boy to this horrible and heartbreaking disease.

*Laura Villeneuve*

# Seth, 11 Years Old

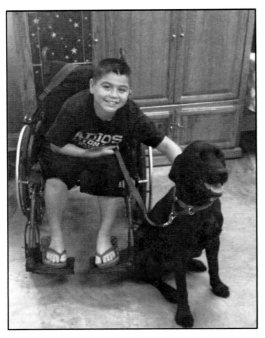

Seth was born on October 17th, 2000. What a wonderful day; we were blessed with a healthy baby boy. I was a stay at home mom to Seth's five siblings, so when we brought Seth home, I spent my days caring for him. We didn't see much difference in Seth as he became a toddler. He was not around other children his age very often but his calves seemed large for a boy his age. He walked on his toes, and the common cold always seemed to end in pneumonia. We would ask the doctors about it, but we were always told that he would grow out of it. What parent wouldn't want their son to have large calve muscles?

Seth was almost six when he started kindergarten. It was hard on us both as he cried for me not to leave him and I cried because he had to go. Soon, Seth began falling at school and no one seemed to know why or how. But it seemed that after each fall he needed to get stitched or stapled. Not once in six years at home with me did this happen, what was going on? Once when Seth had fallen and we went to the clinic, he looked at the doctor and said, "I prefer staples instead of stitches. Can you picture that doctor's face? They didn't have staples, so he got stitched and not one tear was shed. Seth was not able to learn like the other students. This seemed to frustrate his teacher and I became angry with her impatience with Seth. I began attending school whenever possible, and soon switched him into another classroom. His new teacher was better, but Seth's learning abilities were still lacking.

Seth started at a new school in first grade, but the new school brought new problems. Children began picking on Seth because he was different. One day he came home upset after a boy took his lunch box and began hitting him with it. His teacher, a friend of mine, was concerned and was trying to find a solution. This was a nice change. Seth would stare at his journal everyday instead of picking up his pencil and writing like the other kids. One day he took another kid's paper, put his name on it, and turned it in as his own.

Enough was enough; we couldn't keep waiting for him to grow out of it! This time at the doctor's office we demanded options: therapy to stretch his legs, anything to help him. We were referred to an orthopedic specialist and were able to get in the following week. Seth, his 8-month old brother and I went to the appointment. I was excited about getting Seth some help. The doctor had Seth walk down the hall, sit and stand up, and then he looked him over. He looked at me and said that he believed that Seth had Duchenne Muscular Dystrophy (DMD). He briefly explained what DMD was and how to confirm the diagnosis. I tried to reason with him, explaining we were only there to get Seth some physical therapy to help him grow out of this! We left the office and went right to the lab to have Seth's blood drawn to test his protein levels (CPK) and DNA. I tried to smile and stay strong so my boys didn't see that something was wrong.

When I got the boys in the car, I stood outside and began to cry. I called my husband and some other family members, as I was desperately trying to make sense of what had just happened. I got home and began to research Duchenne Muscular Dystrophy. As you read, even though the signs are there, you can't allow yourself to believe it. There is still hope the doctor is wrong. Your heart literally hurts; it is breaking. You pray for something else, anything is better than this diagnosis.

The test results finally came back and Seth's protein levels (CPK) were over 16,000, a normal level is around 250. This confirms that he has DMD.

We waited 6 weeks for his DNA results which showed he was missing exon 51. Only seven years old and we now know that Seth will not grow out of this; things will only get worse from this point on.

Seth was pulled out of school and I began home schooling him. We began going to see several specialists and continued to research treatments online. After much prayer, thought, and conversation, we started Seth on Prednizone in March of 2008. Seth was diagnosed with learning disabilities later that fall. Watching Seth during this time, it seemed he was still a regular boy. It almost felt like the diagnosis of DMD was just a bad dream. There were things that made Seth different, like not being able to lift the gallon of milk, hold his pencil to write, or walk up the stairs without tiring. Those things became normal and we just looked past them. It was easy to put DMD out of our mind until the next doctor appointment or when new information on research became available. Seth was a boy full of life, not knowing DMD was going to change his future. I think from the day Seth was diagnosed we have tried to live every day to the fullest. We've made changes in our lives we may not have made if things were different.

Nothing has prepared us for where we are now, the transition phase. I feel like I woke up one day and BAM DMD just took over. Now we see what DMD is all about; the pain it brings you and all the sadness that comes as your son begins to show the real signs that DMD is here to stay. Seth began falling more, and it became harder for him to walk and easier to just sit. He began asking to be carried upstairs and was less motivated to do things. We ordered Seth a motorized wheelchair in June of 2011. That was a hard and emotional step. I would ask myself, is it really time, is this the right choice, or are we allowing him to give in to the DMD and stop fighting?

In July, Seth and I traveled to GA to train with a service dog. When we came home, we really saw a difference in Seth and his abilities. When the wheelchair was delivered in August, Seth seemed happy about it. Seth is not one to complain and he does not talk much, if at all, about DMD and what it is doing to him. Most of the time I feel he is more concerned about me and how this is impacting me. This phase has been very difficult and overwhelming to say the least.

We have been trying to modify our home to be handicap accessible. This has been such a frustrating experience: building ramps, looking at changing vehicles, and everything else that is needed-for Seth to function. These things are so important because the independence the wheelchair has given him is amazing, but without the ramps and vehicle, his independence is still limited. I spend my time on line or on the phone, only to find there is not much assistance out there and the additional cost to provide these things is astronomical. I try to set my emotions aside so we can conquer each day.

When I look at Seth, I can see and feel that he is on an emotional roller coaster. Things just seem to bother him more lately, his patience is lacking, and he seems angry too often. Seth is now a preteen who does not want my help, but the reality is that he needs it. I think he would rather sit in the restroom and try to figure a way off the toilet than call me for help. He would rather not take that shower because just the thought of it exhausts him and he doesn't want someone in the bathroom with him. I struggle to find the best way to help him deal with DMD and what it is doing to him emotionally and physically.

As I watch my son today, he is wheeling through life instead of walking. I find myself thinking of him finally being able to run like he has always dreamed about. He has back the independence with his wheelchair that DMD robbed him of. I feel uncertain of what tomorrow will bring because DMD is in our life. I know that God has chosen us: Seth, myself, my husband and our family. I'm not sure of the reason, but I know we need to be doing something. I can say for sure that we will be a voice for Seth and the other Duchenne families. We will care for Seth the best we know how. I tell Seth, "I will care for you with all the love in my heart and with a smile on my face, no matter what."

*Kerry Gutierrez*

# Nick, 12 Years Old

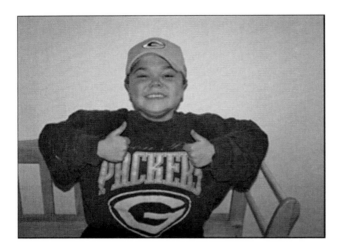

"Dear Duchenne muscular dystrophy, I don't like you. You're kind of a bully; you make people cry. Maybe you should pick up your stuff and go, because you're not really welcome here—none of my friends like you either."

*Gretchen Egner*

# Jackson, 15 Years Old
# and Hayden, 13 Years Old

## (The Dad's Perspective)

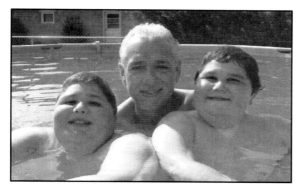

This story is about how my sons changed their daddy. Cynicism has been replaced by compassion; self-pity has turned to hope. Anger still looms over me like a cloud, but that cloud is laced with faith. Unhappiness used to be over not having money or over social injustices, ignorance and sloth. Now I am unhappy that I wasted my time worrying about it. My happiest moments are surrounded by love; I have found that it is not a tangible thing. You cannot measure it, put it in a category, or rank it on a list. You have to feel it. Smiles, a laugh, a hug, a quiet moment spent together, even an argument, can make you feel like a million dollars. A child rising to your defense or remembering what you did or said is worth its weight in gold. Every moment in time becomes precious. Everything you do together in every moment becomes a lasting memory. My sons have saved my life. I only hope that I can return the favor.

## Lucky Man

Yes, I started right off with plagiarism. I was fortunate enough to see Michael J. Fox, who has Parkinson's disease, in person at the Rochester Institute of Technology a couple of months ago. This experience led me to borrowing the title of his book. Most people don't dwell on the subject of death. We struggle with the topic for sure, somewhere in the backs of our minds, but for the most part, we are all too busy to linger on the concept for more than a few moments at a time, unless it is the topic of conversation, such as at a funeral or a will planning appointment with your attorney, where it is still a morbid conversation at best. Death is a topic that is, for the most part, avoided by groups of people. The individual mind is another story entirely. Still, unless you have an unhealthy preoccupation with dying, which would indicate that you are either suffering from a fatal disease, are a funeral director, chief of surgery at a hospital, or psychotic, then like any other normal individual, you don't think about it that much. It is just too depressing.

As for me, it is my constant companion. The ghost of mortality is with me constantly. Not my own mortality, but that of my children. I have a twenty-two year old daughter who is perfectly healthy. I also have two sons with muscular dystrophy. They say that most men lead lives of quiet desperation. I wish this were true; in my case, it is a full-fledged scream. I live daily, with the knowledge that I will probably outlive my sons. Surprisingly, I only ever think about it when I am away from them. The thought never occurs to me when I am with them. I am a part-time dad, and as such, I am away from them a lot. I am told that I have a fifteen-hundred-word limit for my story here. Most men could sum up their experiences with muscular dystrophy in three words, (FIND A CURE!). I find it hard to sum it up in less than thirty thousand!

My boys live with their mom. I have my sons on Tuesdays, Thursdays and one or two Saturdays a month. Because of their special needs, they cannot come to my house. They need the symmetry and structure that is provided by a consistent and stable environment, something that's provided for exceptionally well at their mother's house. So I try to maintain a schedule that allows me to be there on the days that I mentioned, both to promote this stability and to allow their mother to maintain some sort of sanity for herself, as this is her only free time. Obviously, this puts a strain on my ability to hold a job, as I require a work schedule that allows me to be available to my sons on the specified days. However, my attitude toward work has been altered greatly in the last few years. I used to be a man who cared for nothing more than the power and prestige of a demanding job. There was also the issue of the almighty dollar. Sadly, in our world, the American dream has been reduced to a monetary goal. It is no longer about who you are but about what you own. I missed so many holidays and special occasions under the guise of "having to work," that I am ashamed of myself. It took my children to change this. It turns out that I had everything that was important in life already. The day- to-day lifestyle that I lead now has been altered greatly. It is no longer about money. I live for life and love, health and friendship, the true American dream.

I live with a wonderful woman, who supports both me and my new-found ideals. She has three full-grown sons who have children of their own. So I have four surrogate grandchildren, even though my own children are not yet old enough to have children. Well, my daughter Hope is, but fortunately, she is in college and has not had children yet. Not that I don't want her to have them, mind you, I just want her to have them when she is ready. How do I tell my sons that they probably will never be able to raise a family? At any rate, I have four grandchildren already. I have been with my significant other since most of them were born, and I can honestly tell you that they are as much my grandchildren as they are Marilyn's. My favorite was Connor. Yes, I said was. We lost him to childhood cancer, this summer. He was nine. He had my heart strings wrapped around his little finger, just like my own children. He was perfect. Now he's gone. He was a Godsend on Earth, and now he is an Angel in Heaven. My boys, however, are still here; let me tell you about them.

At the time that I am writing this, Jackson is fifteen. His brother, Hayden, is thirteen. For the most part, they are your typical teenage siblings. They fight a lot, they have problems with each other a lot, and yes, they play together a lot. Just like most siblings, though, they have a fierce love for each other that cannot be denied. That being said, my boys are typical for their age group. They hate school, homework, girls (except for their mom, of course), and they hate being idle. On the other side of the coin, they love to be outside, they love to be active, and they love video games. The only difference is that they have to do it from wheelchairs. This presents as many opportunities as it does problems, though. Although my boys need help with normal activities like dressing, personal hygiene, and writing, they enjoy a mobility that others of their age group do not. We can, literally, take a five-mile hike during good weather, without their being bored or tired. Their power-chairs make it necessary for me to ride a bicycle to keep up. One might say that they help me to stay in shape. In fact, between the walks and homework and all of the normal stuff that we have to do, they keep me on my toes. I am busy from the time that I pick them up from school, to the time that I leave at night, and I have the easy end. Their mother has to bathe them, take them to doctors, put them to bed, and really handle anything else that needs to be accomplished. Plus, she has to maintain a household; I don't know how she does it. (I envy her.) There are not enough hours in the day. At any rate, with the exception of the constrictions of a debilitating disease, my sons' lives are pretty much normal.

Both of my boys are sensitive, caring individuals, who love their parents and family and would protect them with their lives. They are smart and funny and all too aware of the disease that holds them hostage. It pains me every minute that we are apart to think of the problems that they will encounter in the future, not for my welfare but for theirs. Yet, I am never aware of that pain, when we are together. Maybe it is because I am too busy to think about it, but I don't believe that this is the case. When I am with my sons, we enjoy each other's' company too much to be sad. Chalk it up too fate or karma or whatever else controls your destiny, but my boys and I enjoy a relationship that includes nothing but quality time. Not a minute is wasted. I can wager that a lot of parents out there are not as lucky. I cherish every joke, every laugh, and every word that is spoken. Even the sarcastic barbs that they hurl at me are sweetened by the knowledge that we are able to share them together, right now. I find myself noticing things that I might otherwise have overlooked, if they were average kids. Their disease has taught me to look at the gifts that make my children special, not the handicaps that make them different.

For example, Jackson, my oldest, is fiercely protective of his brother and his mother. He is compassionate toward everyone and everything, including those less fortunate than he. My knowing what he knows about his condition makes it hard to imagine how he can feel this emotion at all. I am ashamed that I do not live up to his example. Jackson loves to compete at board and video games, and although he likes to win, he can appreciate it when his sister or I beat him at cards or Clue, although we seldom beat him at dominoes. He is sensitive about everything and worries about how he looks to others. He has a God-given talent for music. When he seriously sings a song, he sounds like an angel. He once sang "You are my Sunshine" for his mother and it brought tears to my eyes. He turns sixteen on December 4 and can't wait to drive. How do I tell him that he probably never will?

Hayden was born on June 9, two years after his brother. He is as precocious as they come and shares many of his brother's traits. He is different in many ways, though. Hayden lives in his own world. I really think that he believes he is indigenous to the planet Mars. He has a vivid imagination and a natural affinity towards obsessive behavior. He loves stories and lists. He makes them constantly. He collects things. The best trait of all is his memory. If he sees something once, it is in there forever. One time, when he finished beating a video game, he wrote down a list of every level, sublevel, weapon, and character in the game, from memory! It took four pages. Although he claims to hate reading, it applies only to school. Hayden doesn't talk to you unless you interest him; then you can't shut him up. When we are walking, he must say, "Daddy, remember this," about a thousand times. (I love it.) He is aware of his disease, but not of its outcome. He gets to watch his brother go through it all first with the full knowledge that the same fate awaits him!

I know that what I have written does not begin to explain the hardships that my sons have to live with daily. I also know that what I have said sounds almost cavalier. It kills me every day to think about the past, (the day I became a part-time parent for example.) The future does not look much brighter, (living with the knowledge that I will outlive my sons.) Still, I get to have them right now. We share a relationship that is timeless. We will prevail. As Lou Gehrig said, "On this day I feel that I am the luckiest man, on Earth."

*Robert Alm*

# Jackson, 15 Years Old and Hayden, 13 Years Old

## (The Mom's Perspective)

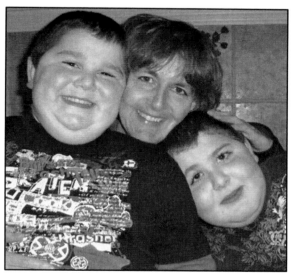

I had reached a point in my life when I thought being a mom was not going to happen for me. I was 35 years old, and neither a short marriage, nor a seven- year relationship had led to children. I started a new relationship but was still not sure I would ever be a mom. When I learned that I was expecting in April of 1994, I was thrilled. I found out that it would be a boy and we named him Jackson Robert Alm. He was perfect! My OB/GYN had said she thought he would be about 7 pounds. When Jackson arrived the doctor looked at everyone and announced, "Someone misjudged this baby!" Jackson was a "healthy" 9 pound 8 ounce baby. I loved being a mom to a beautiful curly haired baby boy. I was a little overwhelmed being 35 years old and a first-time mom. I think I had a touch of postpartum, but he was so much fun.

I noticed fairly early that Jackson was a little slower to reach the milestones than other children his age. He took longer to roll over, sit up, and drink from a cup. Jackson never crawled; he went straight to walking at one year of age. I still did not think anything was wrong because I knew all babies were different. On June 9th, 1998, I gave birth to my second beautiful baby boy. We named him Hayden John Alm. At one year when he was not walking, the pediatrician recommended "early intervention". The early intervention team evaluated Hayden and determined he would benefit from speech, occupational and physical therapies. The therapists came twice each week to our home.

I was working as a professional school bus driver for the town of Greece, NY. Jackson and Hayden were going to daycare while I worked. I started to notice that Jackson had trouble keeping up with the other children. He could barely get up the ladder to the small plastic slide while another boy who was the same age would run up the stairs and jump from the top of the slide to the ground. When Jackson was around four I requested the early intervention team evaluate him as well. They approved him. He started preschool a few months later and on one of Jackson's evaluations the teachers wrote that they noticed "decreased muscle strength" in his legs. The pediatrician then sent us to a neurologist. You never forget the first time you hear the words, "muscular dystrophy". You can feel your heart stop beating and everything feels like it is in slow motion at that point. Then you start to ask questions. Fear is the next emotion you feel. Is there a cure? Are you sure he has this disease? Will he die? I remember leaving the hospital and calling my parents. I was crying and Jackson was just standing next to me not knowing why I was crying. I didn't realize it at the time but the doctors really only need a CPK protein test to determine if a child has Duchenne Muscular Dystrophy (DMD). I remember the doctor saying something about getting a confirmation and finding out about mutations. A muscle biopsy was needed for this so I agreed to have it done. I hated that Jackson had to have anesthesia. There is something horrible about watching your child's eyes roll back in his head.

By this time the boys and I had moved into a small house I had purchased with some help from my parents. You never forget certain moments in this "journey". The moment I was told that here was no doubt that Jackson had DMD was one of those moments for me. I had just dropped the boys off at their dad's house for the weekend. I called the doctor for the results of Jackson's muscle biopsy. I remember just starting to cry in the car. I cried for hours just driving around not sure where I was going. I called friends and we cried together. Then I had to tell my parents. That was one of the hardest things I have ever had to do. My dad always dreamed of a grandson going to Notre Dame. There are so many feelings that you don't expect in this situation. It is the same grieving process for a terminal disease. The steps are the same. I had already done denial before the muscle biopsy.

Next was anger. I bargained with God before the biopsy was done. You promise anything if only it weren't true. Depression then sets in. Every night for weeks I cried myself to sleep. Every morning I woke up and thought it must have been a bad dream.

I started searching the internet for treatments, trials, research, and any kind of hope. That is where I found acceptance. I found so many things happening that gave me hope. Probably the biggest was the fact that children with DMD were living longer than ever before. Twenty to thirty years ago there were very few living past their teens and there were no treatments to speak of. Now boys and a few girls were living well into their 20's and beyond. Some living into their 30's and even 40's! Everything about this disease is so overwhelming. What medications or supplements do you start them one? Are there trials they are eligible for? Where do we go for help with modifications for our homes, for transportation, for support groups? I found networking to be the biggest help, connecting to others who are going through this same struggle.

As the years went on, I seemed to always have a knot in my stomach. If there is any good to DMD, it is that it forces you to see what you are made of. It also makes you so close to your children because you are happy for every moment you have with them. We don't know how much time we have. I have also met some wonderful people that I would never have met otherwise: doctors, physical therapists, occupational therapists, special ed teachers, parents and children with DMD, service coordinators, educational advocates, and countless others. I have had complete strangers touch my arm and tell me they admire me. I took an educational advocate class a few years ago and I remember one of the lecturers saying that we will continue to grieve. When you learn your child has this disease you think of his future. Will your child walk across the stage to get his diploma; will he get married, play sports or have children? You think of all the loss.

The first Muscular Dystrophy Association telethon I was part of, I remember sitting outside on a break and watching some boys play Frisbee and I started to cry. Sometimes I see kids walking along talking and laughing and I feel the tears start again. The challenges for a single mom with two boys with DMD are many. I had hoped that Hayden, my youngest did not have this disease but I guess down deep I knew he did. He had the same tell-tale signs of enlarged calves that Jackson had. He was diagnosed at age four. I am a carrier but we don't know why. My mother is one of nine and it didn't show up anywhere else in her family. Females have a 50/50 chance of being a carrier. There are four sisters in my mother's family and none of their boys had DMD or girls who passed it on to their children. We could have tested my mother but we did not see the point. I informed my entire family that if they were planning on having a family of their own that they might want to get tested for the genetic mutation.

When I found out I was a carrier I thought that I must have done something awful in life to have this happen to me and my boys. Then I realized that God does not punish people by giving a disease to their children. I just could not figure out how this happened. It was silly, but I was just trying to figure out why. This disease is progressive and there is no cure. The muscles weaken more and more over time starting with the legs and then the arms and then on to vital organs such as the heart and lungs. This disease also affects the brain. Many of our boys have learning problems and/or behavior problems. My boys have ADHD and my youngest has OCD, anxiety, selective mutism (he only talks when he wants to), sensory issues, and asthma.

Parents of boys with DMD struggle with decisions about medications like Prednisone, which can make behavior worse and have all kinds of other negative side effects like weight gain, delayed puberty, weakened bones and bloating. I was told that the medication can keep them walking longer though and will help to delay spine surgery which is usually needed later. They may also need heel cord surgery which can be very painful. Other medications like blood pressure or ADHD medications or supplements like Coenzyme CoQ10 (for the heart) are personal choices made by the parents. We have to make decisions about therapies and fight for what we feel they may need in school. We fill out paperwork and call doctors and make appointments with pulmonologists, orthopedists, cardiologists, ADHD doctors, pediatricians, allergists, and schedule sleep study specialists to determine if our boys need a Bi Pap machine to help them breathe better while they are sleeping. We make calls to schools to arrange services our children may need. The good news is that it gets easier after you have been doing it for a while. You learn to get all the medications ordered together, make to do lists, get schedules for appointments, and ask for help whenever you can.

The hardest part of this disease is watching what it does to your child. You watch them start falling and realizing they are different from others their age. Then they lose the ability to walk and have trouble lifting their arms. Next they need machines help them to cough and breathe. Later they may need a tracheotomy to help them breathe. You spend a lot of time comforting your child. I think the second hardest thing besides all the work involved can be judgment from others. I find I get judged for everything from being too happy or too angry to the services we receive from the government. Judgment comes even from family and good friends sometimes. I never want anyone to pity us, but some understanding once in a while would be helpful. I did not have the easiest childhood, including being bullied all through most of my school years, but I cannot even imagine going through what my boys go through each day. They don't get invited to birthday parties and they struggle to find friends. I tell my boys that as much as they have to deal with there are still others who are worse off. It is so hard for a parent to watch her children suffer. When I get tired and feel like I can't go on, I just look at my boys and remember that at least I can walk, eat, brush my teeth and go to the bathroom on my own. I remember a conversation I had with my cousin,

Anne, once. I asked her what made God think I could deal with all this and not put my boys in a home and go to Aruba or something? She told me that she believed God had chosen me to be Jackson and Hayden's mom. I cry when I remember her saying that to me. So that is how I try to think of our journey. We were chosen by God to be together.

I will continue to help my boys through their anger and frustration with hugs and kisses and laughter. I will make them comfortable at night when they need their braces and leg wedges, and their legs tied together with a robe tie so they don't fall to the side. And I will keep using my monitor to listen when they call me in the middle of the night to straighten a leg or take off a brace that is hurting. I will watch for new breakthroughs and new trials that may work for my boys. We will continue to cry and to laugh like when we are in public bathrooms that are too small and we just laugh at ourselves while we try to make it work. I will continue to yell about anything I see out in the public that is not accessible and things my boys need. I will continue to pray that something will come along to at least keep my boys alive longer than expected. And I will continue to do whatever it takes to make my boys feel loved and accepted forever.

*Diane M Keeley*

# Benjamin, 15 Years Old
## and Samuel, 13 Years Old

### A Journey of Faith

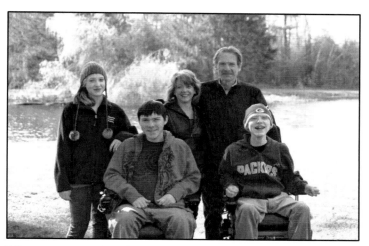

Like so many other families, our journey has been one of faith. On May 27, 2002, at 8:15 p.m. as we were reading bedtime Bible stories, our home was struck by lightning. For the 12 weeks it took to repair the resulting fire and water damage, we lived in a hotel. In early June at Benjamin's 6th year check-up, our family doctor agreed to a PT/Orthopedic referral, because Ben was constantly walking on his toes, struggling to walk up stairs, and not able to keep up with his peers. I must give my mom credit for pushing me to have Ben checked by a specialist. Mike and I had been thinking he would eventually catch up to everyone else. How wrong we were!

A genetic test was ordered a few weeks later. Mike, who was working full-time and traveling a lot, took Ben into Boston for that appointment. I stayed home with Sam and Lydia, who were 4 and 3 at the time. My loving husband never told me that muscular dystrophy might be a possible diagnosis. I think he was trying to protect me from 4 weeks of worry and heartbreak awaiting the DNA results.

On August 7th while the kids and I were trying to nap, Mike called from work with the devastating news that Benjamin's DNA test had come back positive for Duchenne Muscular Dystrophy (DMD). Although I was lying in bed with all 3 children at the time, I couldn't even pretend to hide my pain. The cries came from deep within my soul and the tears were endless. My entire life changed in that moment. It was as if all of my hopes and dreams for my son had been shattered into a million pieces.

As I tried to make sense out of it all over the next few days, I spent much time on the Internet. To my horror, I learned that a wheelchair wasn't 10 or 12 years down the road, but by age 10 or 12. Then I read those awful words, "Life expectancy is rare past the late twenties." How could my great, loving, all-powerful God be allowing this to happen to my child...to me? As I grieved those first few days and weeks, I felt as if my insides were being ripped out. On the morning of August 12th I was praying in the bedroom while Lydia slept and the boys played in the living room. When I finished, I came out with a smile on my face but Benjamin said, "Mommy, I heard you crying while you were praying." As I took my beautiful little boy on my lap and held him close I said, "Benjamin, some things in life are very sad, but as long as you trust Jesus, you will have joy in the midst of sadness."

After breakfast, we sat down to read, *Keys for Kids*, a children's devotional. The key verse was John 11:35, "Jesus wept." As my children and I read about how Jesus cried when He saw the pain of others at Lazarus's death, I knew that Jesus understood and felt my pain. He would be with me and carry me through this trial. Nothing, not muscular dystrophy or anything else this life has in store for me, could ever make me doubt the love of God. I prayed furiously that Samuel and Lydia would be spared, but that was not God's plan. On August 16th Samuel was also diagnosed with DMD and we learned that our precious Lydia carried the genetic defect. You may think this strange, but I had the hardest time with Lydia's diagnosis. Not only was I mourning the eventual loss of my boys, but I was mourning the loss of ever becoming a grandmother as well.

By now our lightning-damaged home was ready to move back into. My family pitched in with the kids while I cleaned the house, made beds and unpacked every item we owned. I was grateful for the many times my father-in-law came down to watch the kids for me during this time. One night Mike and I went out for dinner alone while my sister had the kids and I felt closer to him than I had in a very long time. Maybe this horrible disease would bring our family closer together. It certainly was bringing me closer to God.

One of the deepest prayers of my heart was that God would bring someone alongside me who could understand what I was going through. Everyone else I knew had typical children and although some of them tried, family members and friends couldn't relate to my pain. A series of events that only God could orchestrate led me to my dear friend Joan Lafferty. She has been a blessing in my life from the very first time I called her. Her story also appears in this book.

That fall I homeschooled Ben and loved snuggling together on the couch reading and working on math, phonics and handwriting. Around this time our pastor preached a message on Abraham and Isaac. I wept through the entire message as I listened to how God had called Abraham to sacrifice his one and only son. I thought about how God was asking me to let go of Ben and Sam, two of the most precious people in my life. Why God? And then I wept even more when I remembered that God Himself had sacrificed His one and only Son so that whoever believes in Him might be saved (John 3:16).

I think I cried every time I was in church those first few months after the diagnosis. As I write this, we have just observed the 10th anniversary of 9/11. Like most of you, our family spent several days watching television coverage and listening to radio broadcasts from the survivors of that horrific attack. One message kept coming through loud and clear: *tragedies like 9/11 reveal both the best and the worst in humankind.* As I contemplated the sheer evil behind those attacks and the true heroism of the victims and first responders, I couldn't help comparing it to DMD. People's lives changed in an instant on 9/11 just like ours did when we were given the diagnosis. Tragedies like 9/11 and Duchenne bring out the best and the worst in our friends, families, and even strangers. Some people break our hearts and walk away, not knowing how to journey down this road with us. Others bless us in amazing ways!

As the shock of the diagnosis started to wane, Duchenne became like a cloud that enveloped me wherever I went. I was in a constant state of sadness. I started to fast and pray to God for a miracle, but also to prove to Him that I would be faithful whatever His will might be for Ben and Sam. As time went on, I realized that God's plan was not to cure Ben and Sam, but to use them for His glory. Knowing that God can and will use even DMD to reveal Himself through Ben and Sam has been a huge comfort to me.

Although I was doing my best to trust God, I struggled with a passage of Scripture in the Book of Psalms. Psalm 139 says that God covers us in our mother's womb and that we are "fearfully and wonderfully" made. How could Ben and Sam have been *wonderfully* made since they have a fatal genetic disease? If you ask God something with an open heart, He will eventually answer you. Two years after Ben and Sam's diagnosis, I heard a message on Psalm 139 and learned that in the original Hebrew language "fearfully" means "*to inspire reverence and godly fear*"; "wonderfully" means "*separated or set apart*". It was as if a light bulb turned on in my head: God had created Ben and Sam with a purpose, to be separated and set apart for Him! God makes no mistakes. It was no accident that Ben and Sam have Duchenne. God allowed the genetic mutation and He was going to use it.

So much has happened in the ensuing years. We built an accessible home and purchased a full-size wheelchair van and all kinds of adaptive equipment. My step-dad was so gracious to build a wheelchair ramp onto their home without ever being asked. It is such a blessing to have another home that is accessible to our family. My brother and sister took my boys up to my uncle's camp in the White Mountains when it was too difficult for me to do it anymore. Ben and Sam both recently received their second power wheel-chairs and they are now using respiratory equipment as well. We have been to hundreds of appointments with physical therapists, physiatrists, neurologists, cardiologists, pulmonologists, orthopedic surgeons and more. Ben has had hamstring and hip flexor tendon releases and a complete spinal fusion surgery. Although we opted to skip the tendon releases on Sam, he will most likely endure the 10-hour spinal fusion surgery and 12-week recovery at the end of this school year.

But it has not all been hardship and pain. We have seen God's hand of blessing over and over again. Although he lived for only 10 months after we received the devastating diagnosis, I watched my dad's heart soften so much in that short time. We have also met some incredible people and have done some amazing things over the past 9 years. The boys have enjoyed adaptive snow and water skiing and we are currently looking into a local Power Soccer league. They both enjoyed an amazing trip to Florida with Make-A-Wish. All 3 children have been ambassadors for Make-A-Wish at local fundraising events. Sam is currently taking drum lessons from a man with BMD and all of my children sing in a Christian youth choir. Last year at our church's Thanksgiving testimony service, I was finally able to publically admit that the blessings of DMD far outweigh the pain and that God has used these trials to make me a better person than I ever would have been without them.

This past summer I had an incredible experience with a group of ladies called *Gals for Cal*. It started when I attended an MDA support group meeting and met a man named Dave whose wife had done a triathlon to benefit The Jett Foundation. My ears perked up because the thought of doing a triathlon before I turned 50 had been in the back of my mind. Soon I was signed up with 8 other DMD moms and a group of friends and family members (85 in total) to do a sprint triathlon. I hadn't been on a bike in almost 20 years and I had never really learned to swim. I signed up for lessons with the swim coach at my gym, got my old mountain bike tuned up, bought a new pair of running sneakers and I was off! The camaraderie, fun, and feeling of empowerment as we raised over $43,000 for the Jett Foundation were unbelievable. As an added benefit, Ben and Sam were able to attend Camp Promise East, a camp for kids with neuromuscular diseases, which was totally funded by The Jett Foundation.

We have also had an amazing time attending Joni and Friends Family Retreats for people with disabilities. What a joy to be in a place with hundreds of other people who just "get it". They have a wonderful sibling group run by a college-aged student who has a teenage brother with cognitive disabilities. Lydia loves getting together with other teens and pre-teens that have siblings with disabilities. Even though caring for our affected sons is often exhausting, we must make time to meet the needs of our typical children as well. For the past several years I have had the privilege of co-leading a Joni and Friends moms group where I live in New Hampshire. Even though our children's ages and disabilities are varied, we are able to understand and comfort one another because God has led us on similar journeys. One of my favorite Bible passages is 2 Corinthians 1:3-7: "Blessed be God…who comforts us in all our trouble, so that we can comfort (others) with the comfort we ourselves have received from God…We know that just as you share in our sufferings, so you also share in our comfort." My message to those of you living the nightmare of DMD is this: "Don't waste even one moment of the pain and suffering you are enduring. If you are willing, God will use you to serve and minister to others like no one else can". And my message to friends and family members is: "Don't be afraid to enter into our pain. If you reach out of your comfort zone and find ways to serve and help those of us living this nightmare, you will be blessed beyond measure."

Even small gestures like giving Lydia a ride home from volleyball practice so I don't have to load and bring both Ben and Sam to pick her up are a huge blessing to me. My children attend a small Christian school and we have been blessed by the staff and even some students who help Ben and Sam with everything from toileting to sharpening pencils during the school day. There are times when I see friends helping them pack up their books or perform some other activity and my heart is warmed. Ben was asked to be the score keeper for the soccer team and has done that for several years. Being included on the team even though he cannot play has been very important to Ben. This past year he was asked by our pastor to be an usher and he has faithfully done that with joy ever since.

There have also been times over the years when people have been unknowingly inconsiderate or unkind in their words and actions. Over the many weeks following Ben's spinal fusion surgery, he received only two short visits from classmates. That was very hurtful to all of us. There have also been times when my boys have not been included in sleepovers, birthday parties, and other activities. It is difficult to watch my teen boys becoming more and more dependent while their friends become more and more independent. But my hope is that we are all able to see past a disability to the actual heart of a person and know that they too want to be needed, accepted and loved. Whenever I start to become discouraged and disappointed in people, I'm stopped when I remember how oblivious I was to the needs of people with disabilities before I was thrown into this world myself. As much as I'd like to believe that I would always be helpful and never be hurtful to someone else going through a tragedy like this, the fact is that I am only a sinner saved by grace and I need to extend that grace to others.

Just as that hotel was merely a temporary residence for us while our home was being repaired, this world is only a stepping stone into eternity for each one of us. We must all be ready to meet our Maker. God never promised us an easy life on this earth, but His Word tells us that in heaven there will be no more sorrow, no more tears and absolutely NO more wheelchairs! I eagerly await that day.

*Lori Safford*

## *Lydia Safford, Sister of Ben and Sam, age 12*
### *The Pain of Being a Sibling*

Hey my name is Lydia, and I have 2 brothers in wheelchairs that have muscular dystrophy and I'm also a carrier. Yes, sometimes it's really hard and I get depressed because of it. But my brothers also inspire me a lot. And we have really good times, and I'm glad because one day they won't be here to have them. It gets hard for me sometimes because I have to do a lot of things around the house that my brothers can't do. But I love them so much and I know that one day I'll see them in heaven.

# Hurricane, 16 Years Old

## *I Would Choose You in a Heartbeat*

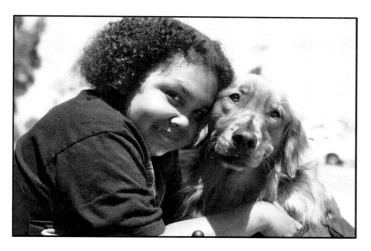

## *I Wanted Him to Die*

I'd always been an upbeat, positive person. I greeted each day with a bright smile and words of inspiration. Then, after May 4, 2001, I thought I would never smile again. On that day my five-year old son, Hurricane, was diagnosed with Duchenne Muscular Dystrophy.

When they told me this muscle wasting disease, for which there is yet no cure, would slowly rob my precious child of all muscle capacity, I wanted him to die. When they said it would not only affect his arms and legs, but his heart and his lungs and all the areas that keep him alive, I wanted him to die immediately. All I could imagine for him was a life of limitation, frustration, loneliness, fear, and suffering. That's all that I could imagine, and I wanted no part of it.

These are thoughts and feelings I am not proud of.

Many of you, in your compassion for me, are immediately thinking I simply did not want my son to suffer. What mother would? While that is certainly true, it was not the primary reason I wanted him to die. My primary reason was completely selfish; I did not want to *watch* him suffer.

As parents, we instinctively desire to keep our children safe. We want to protect them from as many hardships as we can. I don't believe, however, we want to spare them life's trials and tribulations for purely altruistic reasons; we are really trying to save ourselves the anguish of watching our beloveds endure those hardships. The love we have for our children connects us to them in a very intimate and special way. When they cry, we cry as well. When they suffer, we suffer. When they feel pain, we feel it too. It seems we feel it to the same degree, if not more so. We really want to spare our children that pain in order to spare ourselves. At least that is how it was for me.

In the five years I had the privilege of having this beautiful child in my life, my love for him had expanded exponentially. I never knew I could love someone so much. Before I had children, I surveyed various parents to get a better understanding of what I was about to get into. They all spoke of a love so vast, so deep it was impossible to describe. I thought they were nuts. It could not possibly be that great, that intense. Then I had Hurricane and knew they were right. I had Hurricane and I understood.

My love for Hurricane started long before he was born. It started when his name was chosen and continued as my husband Mark and I contemplated conception for three years. The love leaped forward when I first saw his heartbeat in the doctor's office and it grew every day as he matured inside my body. When he was born, the love fully blossomed. Every day thereafter, my love for this precious baby grew and grew. I sometimes thought my heart would actually explode if I loved him anymore. And then I would love him twice as much as I did the week before.

At five years old, when Hurricane was diagnosed with DMD, my love was just five years deep, and it was all consuming. I knew with every year he continued to live I would only love him more. Thus, I imagined whenever the end came, the hurt I would feel would be more than I could stand. I concluded that watching what was likely to happen to my son would be just too much for me to bear. Every time I thought about it I would have trouble breathing, get lightheaded and want to throw up.

So I wanted it to end right then. I wanted him to die. It was an ugly, frightening thought and I was ashamed of it, yet I could not get rid of it. I spoke of it to no one, not my husband, not my girlfriends, no one. How could I explain this terrible selfish thought? How would I defend myself against the reprimands I imagined people would have for me? Instead, I buried this unspeakable thought deep inside where it haunted me, day in and day out, during my waking hours and during my sleep. It haunted me until I dreamed it had come true.

## The Dream

The ship bounced gently up and down in the middle of the vast blue ocean. Mark, Hurricane, and I were enjoying the view when we heard screaming and yelling. Something was happening to the ship and suddenly we, along with hundreds of other passengers, were violently tossed into the ocean. We woke up to find ourselves, and the pieces of our broken ship, scattered along the shore of an island.

As soon as I opened my eyes I could see Mark but not Hurricane. Panic took over as I ran around looking for him, asking everyone, "Have you seen my son? Have you seen Hurricane?" No one had seen him. I ran out into the ocean and began swimming, looking for him. And then I found him. I found his body . . . floating face down in the water. I pulled him to shore and I did everything I could to revive him, but he would not breathe. My heart was breaking with every passing moment he failed to respond.

"Come on baby, please, please breathe. Oh God, please let him breathe!"

Panic gave way to hysteria as I began screaming, "No, no, don't take my baby, I want my boy to live; I want him to live!"

Through my screaming and crying, I heard Mark call my name, "Star! Star!"

I opened my eyes to find myself sitting up in my bed in the middle of the night. I had been screaming and crying out loud while I was dreaming. When I looked around and realized it was a dream, I began crying anew. Visibly startled and concerned, Mark tried to calm me down. "What is it, love?" he asked.

"I dreamt Cane died."

Mark held me as I told him my horrid dream. By the time I was through we were both in tears. "Should I go get him to sleep with us?" he asked.

I merely nodded for fear that speaking would restart the torrent of tears. Mark brought our sleeping boy into our bed and placed him between us. I went to sleep that night with my hand on Hurricane's back, comforted by his slow and easy breathing. Relieved my boy was still alive, I drifted off to sleep knowing without a shadow of a doubt I wanted every second I had with Hurricane, no matter what it looked like. I wanted my son to live.

I wanted my son to live so I could enjoy the gift that he is. I wanted him to live so he could enjoy the benefits of life. I wanted him to live so he would know happiness, joy, laughter, sunshine, Disneyland, and cotton candy. I wanted him to live so he would know what it feels like to be loved beyond compare, so he would know what it feels like to see his parents' faces light up at the very sight of him. I wanted him to live.

In the light of a new day, I shifted my focus from the end to the present, from darkness to light, from pain to joy, and from fear to gratitude. In doing so, I was able to move forward with my life and enjoy what really mattered.

It's been 10 years. Hurricane is a beautiful, sweet, smart, funny 15- year old boy. He is also extremely sarcastic and sometimes annoying – everything a teenager should be. Despite some hard times and challenging moments, the past 10 years have been filled with incredible joy, laughter and more love than I could have imagined. Loving Hurricane has blessed my life and made me a better person – more patient, more compassionate; more upbeat and positive than ever before. I wish with all my heart he did not have DMD, but as I told Hurricane one evening when he was about 11 years old.

"If I had a choice between you with DMD or some other boy, I would choose you in a heartbeat."

*Star Bobatoon*

# Joey, 20 Years Old

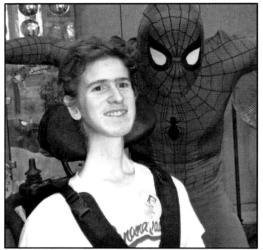

As I am writing this story about Joey, I realize that I didn't want this to be just a story about Joey's suffering, the hardships of raising a sick child, or the heartache. Those things are a part of our lives, but I mostly wanted to give everyone a small glimpse into the heart of Joey. He has never worried much about himself, but; instead, is usually happy and thinking about others.

Joey was born prematurely, January 3, 1991. I will always believe my husband's prayers carried our son through the following days, as Joey fought to live. Due to a fever I had, the nursery would not let me see my son until he was a week old. So his dad was the one who had to go see him, get pictures for me, hold him, and tell him how much we all loved him. Joey fought a good fight. The doctors and hospital staff did an awesome job, and God answered Jeff's prayers.

Joey came home, tiny. He was on a monitor to let us know if his heart stopped or if he stopped breathing. We woke many nights to alarms, only to find Joey perfectly fine, with his little toes tangled in the wires he had managed to kick loose, setting off all the alarms and getting the entire house out of bed in a panic. He grew so fast that my dad accused me of putting Miracle Grow in his formula. Soon, it was hard to believe he had ever been a premature baby.

Doctors warned us that his development might be delayed, so we didn't think much about it when he walked funny or fell down once in a while. We were assured that he would outgrow it. From the time he was three until he was old enough to go to school, a special ed teacher came to the house a couple of times a week.

Joey got into everything he could with his three sisters, Amber, Joanne, and Amanda, but mostly with Joanne. Joanne was the closest in age to Joey, only 14 months younger than he. Looking back now, I believe that she, even as a little child, always understood more than any of us that Joey would need help. Everywhere they went, she was holding his hand and helping him. They have always had a special bond that the rest of us were never part of. Just a few weeks ago, we were moving across the country. Joanne made the trip with me to assist with Joey while we traveled. Since it was raining, I parked at a store and ran inside to buy an umbrella. While I was gone, a man pulled up beside our van, parking too close for us to get the lift down. The next thing I knew, I saw Joanne darting in the store, confronting a stranger, and sending him back outside in the rain to move his car. I will always believe God sent Joanne to be there for Joey all these years.

When Joey was eight, teachers thought he was autistic. So we set appointments to have him tested. Those tests came back fine, but an intern noticed something that everyone had missed over the years. She told us he had Gower's sign. We waited until that afternoon to see a specialist, who told us he suspected Duchenne, but it would be a couple of months before we had a full diagnosis. I went home that night, and like any mom with the Internet, I researched. I knew in the pit of my stomach that everything I read described my son. That day our lives were turned upside down.

A few weeks later, I was home alone with the kids. The phone call came confirming our worst fears. Joey had DMD. One doctor told us he would probably never live to see 20. Joey celebrated his twentieth birthday this past January 3, 2011, and I plan to enjoy many more with him.

The day that I got Joey's diagnosis, Jeff was at work and I didn't want to call and tell him over the phone, so I called my parents. They lived close by, and Dad came as soon as I called. He spent the afternoon with me. My Dad was always the biggest kid in the room when he was with my children. That day was no different. He laughed and played, gave Joey blow kisses on the neck, counted his ribs to make him giggle, and did anything else he could to make him squeal. I sat there thinking to myself, "How can you laugh and have fun right now?" I was a little furious with him; then it hit me! Daddy was right. We had to keep making Joey's life as happy as possible. We needed to laugh and have fun.

Over the years, Joey has had an extraordinary life. He has been to Disneyland, California Land, and to New York City to see the Statue of Liberty and the world's largest Toys R Us in Times Square. Make A Wish sent us all to Orlando to stay at Give Kids the World Village and go to Disney World, Sea World, and his favorite, Universal Studios. He has been Grand Marshall in the Christmas Parade! We also traveled to Sao Paulo, Brazil, to try a treatment there. That was his first plane ride. As the plane went down the runway, Joey was in his seat chanting, "Go Plane, Go Plane!" Joey has been in Special Olympics Bowling, Track and, of course, the Special Olympics Dances, where he was on the dance floor in his power chair dancing with all the girls he could.

Joey grew up very much outnumbered by three sisters. Amber is his older sister. Joanne and Amanda are younger. Joey and Joanne made a daily habit of pulling the top mattress off the bed and dumping it on the floor to turn the entire room into one big trampoline. They would jump off the box springs onto the mattress. That was when Joey wasn't climbing to the top of his closet or getting stuck in the chest of drawers he climbed into after pulling all the drawers out. He certainly kept me on my toes when he was younger!

Over the years, my son has not cried much over his illness. He took it better than most adults when he stopped walking and faced surgeries. While recovering from a tendon release operation, Joanne was in Joey's room checking on him, and she told him how bad she felt because he had to have surgery. His reply was, "Why I only had surgery," like it was no big deal. Joey took his spinal fusion just as well, refusing to cooperate with being ventilated just a few hours after surgery. He wanted the device off, so they had to lessen his pain meds so he could breathe without it. The next morning he insisted on sitting up in a chair. The doctor was amazed. He rarely complained while healing. I think his biggest disappointment was not being able to feed himself anymore.

Just a couple of months later, when our friend's little girl had to have heart surgery, Joey got upset then. He cried and told me he didn't want her not to be able to walk. I assured him that what she had would not make her stop walking. He was concerned about her not walking, but never about himself not walking! Joey had the same concern when his older sister, Amber, was having our first grandbaby, Kaiden.

Every night Joey tells me, "Goodnight" and "I love you." If he thinks I didn't hear him, he calls me back to his room to be sure I got the message! He has the sweetest heart and is the happiest child I have.

Over the years of my life, Joey has been my biggest blessing. He is truly a gift from God above, and we have all learned so much from him. I have never regretted bringing him in this world, as I firmly believe that this world is a better place for having him. I don't worry about the suffering that Duchenne has brought him or us, as everyone has to make the most out of whatever life gives each of us. Joey has certainly made the most of his life and ours too! I know all my girls are better people for having a brother with special needs. At times, they have each had to be second to Joey and his needs, but not one of them has ever complained. Amanda, my youngest, was telling me about a discussion at her school, about what if the people whom we classify as perfect are really the imperfect ones and the ones whom we worry about having problems are really the perfect ones.

I pray we get to keep Joey much longer than predicted. We are now using a treatment called VECTTOR that is giving us and others some very promising results, but I know that no matter the outcome, we are all blessed with each and every day we have him.

*Brenda Morea*

# Eddie, 20 Years Old

## We Live By Hope

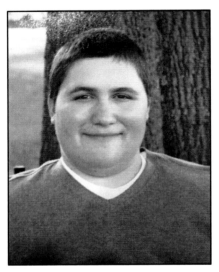

Eddie was our first child, born five weeks premature. His sister, Maggie, was born thirteen months later. The two were inseparable and grew into precocious and inquisitive toddlers. By the time Eddie was two years old, I knew that something was not right. He couldn't run well or jump, and had difficulty getting up from the floor. Maggie was passing him in all of these milestones and was stronger physically. After almost two years of doctor visits and endless medical tests, it was the results of a simple blood test that threw Eddie, and our family, into the clutches of neuromuscular diseases. More tests and a muscle biopsy confirmed our worst nightmare. "Your son has Duchene Muscular Dystrophy (DMD)," we were told by a neurologist, who had told me just the previous week that I "was being an overprotective mother," and that "Eddie probably has delayed gross motor skills due to being a premature baby." This same doctor now could barely look us in the eye; his own eyes glistened with tears as he delivered this devastating news. "Take your son home and love him unconditionally. He will not live a long life." Eddie was two months shy of his fourth birthday.

The diagnosis was completely out of the blue. There is no family history, no genetic or hereditary links. "A spontaneous mutation," we were told. "A fluke". One of the first thoughts that came to my mind was The Jerry Lewis Telethon. My son was now going to be "one of Jerry's kids."

Eddie and his younger sister were too young to understand, but as parents, we quickly came to understand the enormity of a dark cloud enveloping our lives, throwing us into the land of illness that would change our lives, our dreams, and test our faith and our family structure tremendously. We watched more intently and began to notice the physical differences, not just between our own two children, but between Eddie and his peers. Subtle signs became more apparent. We were devastated.

After the initial shock and devastation of hearing this news, we realized we had two choices. We could sit back, do nothing, and let the disease take over our lives. OR we could fight back by doing what we could to raise awareness and funds for research that were so desperately needed. It was an easy choice! We committed ourselves to advocacy. Although we did not realize it at the time of our decision, our pledge to become advocates was not opposed to our commitment to ourselves. In fact, we know now that becoming public advocates actually enhanced our capacity to provide for our son. On our journey from emotions to advocacy, we have learned so much and have met so many caring and wonderful people. We have learned to use our emotions as a source of energy and power. It kept us focused on getting what was needed for our son so he could maintain his independence, health and quality of life.

Our goal became to provide Eddie a life of normalcy within the confines of his disease. It was inevitable that our future was going to revolve around this disease, and we had to integrate it into our lives. It had to become part of his identity. We needed to help him develop his sense of self that enhanced his disability, rather than let it identify him. Planning is essential when dealing with a disability. We had to plan for a future that would ultimately include wheelchairs, elevators, mechanical devices, personal care givers, and breathing and cough machines. Climbing stairs for Eddie became like scaling Mt. Everest on a daily basis. It would have been easier to move to a one-floor ranch home, but we thought the physical location of our home could offer so much to Eddie in fostering his independence. We opted to stay and build an addition that is completely handicap accessible. Playing an active role in providing the best quality of life for Eddie is probably one of the most important and loving gifts we have given him. We made it our mission to be our child's advocate every step of the way. We have used our emotions as a source of energy and power to keep us focused on getting what is needed for him.

When Eddie was in kindergarten, we started our life-long journey as advocates for our son and other children suffering from DMD. We began working with the schools and within the community to promote awareness and raise funds for research. We became advocates for the MDA, forming a team of supporters, including family, friends, neighbors, schoolmates, community members, local businesses and even strangers, who became known as "Eddie's Team". Eddie's Team supported our cause and helped raise over $200,000 for DMD research. We engaged in selling brownies and lemonade, scooping ice cream, and we put on kickathons, hopathons, bike rides and an annual walkathon for eight years; it didn't matter what we did, as long as we were doing something. We have learned that it takes only a few minutes to educate people about the disease, the importance of raising funds for research and how our children have dreams just like their children.

Knowledge is power. We used it to help people understand the urgency that families affected by neuromuscular diseases face every day. These events became a symbol of hope for us and energized us to get through another year.

Our intuition guided us to disclose information to Eddie about his illness slowly, in small doses that he could grasp and understand. In the beginning, we told him that his muscles were weak and he might find it hard keeping up with others. We kept information age- appropriate and vague at a young age, offering more glimpses into the disease process as he got older and began experiencing expected symptoms of the disease. We never discouraged him from doing or trying anything. He played little league and soccer. He skied, skateboarded, and rode a bicycle. He was unyielding in his relentless pursuit to be a "normal" child. However, as the disease progressed, he became more aloof and distanced himself when he couldn't do what the others were doing. A disease or illness can take away that typical enthusiasm of youth that is found in growing children. He was confined to a wheelchair at age ten, and while the wheelchair is a symbol of dependence to some, to the user, it is a source of freedom and independence. He spirits lifted with his new-found freedom, and he was free from the fear and humiliation of falling or being left behind.

Transitioning to middle school brought Eddie new challenges due to his being in a power wheelchair. An inaccessible building and multiple surgeries forced him to miss most of the seventh grade. While the school staff did what they could to accommodate Eddie, it was not enough. Without funding, the school was not in position to build an elevator for accessibility to the entire building. The other middle school in town was accessible, but going there would have taken Eddie away from all of his friends that he had gone to school with since kindergarten. We took matters into our own hands. While Eddie was recuperating from three surgeries in a six-month time period, his father recruited volunteers from the Mass Laborers Union Local 223 and secured enough material donations to build that elevator themselves! Every weekend, for an entire year, "Eddie's Team" of Laborers worked tirelessly, and by the time Eddie returned to school to start eighth grade, the elevator was completed. Today, that elevator is used by many disabled others who came after Eddie.

Dances, proms, college applications, and graduation were the highlights of high school years. Eddie sailed through his studies, achieving high honors while seemingly accepting the progression of his disease and the impact on his body. Graduation was bittersweet; the excitement of achieving that milestone was mixed with fear of leaving the comforts and security of high school and lifelong friends.

Today, Eddie is 20, and is enrolled in a liberal arts program at a local college. He compensates for the frailty of a weakening body by keeping his mind sharp. He is quiet and unassuming, comfortable only in conversation with family and close friends. Even that comes with difficulty sometimes, with shyness and self-consciousness more obstacles to overcome. He is an avid reader, loves going to Boston Bruins hockey games, and playing video games. Ask him about rock music, history, geography, food and he will talk openly and fluently. It's his disease process he won't talk about. He carries the burden of not wanting to talk about a subject that will make his family feel any sadder than they already are. Disability can be a lonely place. One can be afraid to go out of their comfort zone and take risks. People have a tendency to judge based on the disability and not look at the person. Fears surrounding how others are going to treat you and see you are painful, especially at a young age. While his peers are immersed in college life and planning for their futures, Eddie lives a life of anticipating problems and difficulties and has to always plan to avoid mistakes that could get him in trouble. His dreams and goals of going into the military after high school have been abandoned. Fortunately, technology and social media have allowed him to stay connected to old and new friends.

Throughout the years, we have brought countless numbers of people together working towards a common cause, and most importantly, have shown our children that anyone and everyone has the power to make a difference. This has been the gift of advocacy. We have empowered ourselves and our children in the process of expressing our needs, raising money and creating awareness. All it took was strong conviction, a little effort, and hope.

Perhaps the most powerful lesson in all of this is that you have to maintain a human capacity for optimism in spite of the possibility, or even the certainty, of pain and death. In terminal illness, hope represents the patient's and the family's imagined future, forming the basis of a positive, accepting attitude and providing their life with meaning, direction and optimism. When hope is viewed this way, it is not limited to cure of the disease, but focuses on what is achievable in the time remaining. We live life to the fullest, creating a lifetime of memories. Our faith has been strongly tested along the way, fracturing a family unit to the point of depression, separation and near divorce. Disability changes the dynamics of the family. Years of counseling, both individual and family, have helped us all grow, love, and reconnect. It has taught us to understand the dance of anger, denial, and acceptance. Denial can be liberating because it throws off despair and makes all things possible in the time we are given. While we cannot promise our son a quantity of life, his quality of life is immeasurable. We believe strongly that there will be a cure for DMD; our fear is that it may not come soon enough. For today we have hope, but hope doesn't make the pain and the fear go away. We are held captive by DMD and find it difficult to focus on, or plan for, the future. We have to anticipate and plan every day and live for the day we have now. We are making a lifetime of memories in a short period, which is bittersweet in that we are enjoying our time as a family, without the benefit of having time. We live by Hope.

*Margie Saliba*

# Luke, 20 Years Old

## *He is Alive*

*(Excerpt from Celebrating 365 Days of Gratitude, December 22)*

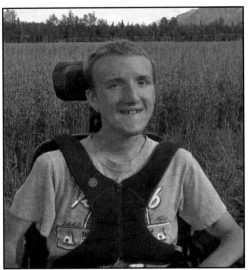

Duchenne Muscular Dystrophy, how can I be grateful for you? You have ravaged my son's body, confining him to a wheelchair, and you have ripped my heart out more times than I can count. That's easy. My soul is singing with gratitude because my son graduated from high school when they told me he probably wouldn't, and he has the diploma to prove it. He escaped having a tracheotomy. He jumped courageously at the chance for healing when others said it was snake oil.

I am grateful for the "firsts" we have celebrated this year –like witnessing him hugging his sister and his health and vitality improving instead of declining. He is taking ahold of the reins of his life when I never thought he'd get the chance. He has given me hope and inspiration to live my purpose on a mission to fight for a cure. He is thriving, not just surviving. Today is his birthday, and he is alive.

*Misty VanderWeele*

Hi my name is Jenna and I am 12 years old. I am Luke's sister. My mom asked me the following questions about my brother since I get very sensitive about my brother.

Mom: What is the most important to you about Luke?
Jenna: That he loves me.

Mom: What do you want others to know about your brother?
Jenna: He is a person not a wheelchair.

Mom: What is your favorite dream you have about Luke?
Jenna: To have him be able to walk with me on the beach.

Mom: What have you learned from your brother?
Jenna: Always be yourself.

Mom: If there was anything you could say to Luke what would that be?
Jenna: I love you just the way you are.

# Adam, 26 Years Old

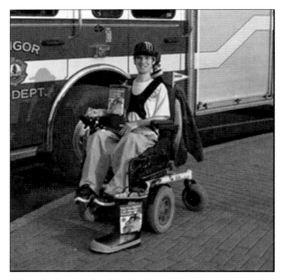

Adam's life started out with a battle because he was born 3 months early.

Adam was born at 29 weeks gestation at home while we were stationed at Royal Air Force Lakenheath, England. A premature home birth was certainly not planned. He spent time in the Wroxham Baby Intensive Care Ward at the Norwich Norfolk Hospital and had surgery when he was only nine days old to close a blood vessel between his heart's aorta and his pulmonary artery. This blood vessel usually closes in the first few days after birth, (Ductus - Arteriosus Closure). He also stopped breathing several times while he was in the Intensive Baby Ward., Adam was later transferred back to the base hospital after gaining weight; he weighed only 2lbs. 14 ozs. when he was born. On Thanksgiving Day we went to visit our little Adam only to see an empty incubator. Instead, he was on the critical baby cart after liquid from a tube feeding aspirated into his lungs. One memory that came back from this episode was when they were poking him with needles to find a spot to insert an IV line. Little Adam cried and we heard him cry for the very first time. Before this, you could tell he was crying from his facial expression, but his lungs were too weak and we weren't able to hear the crying sounds.

As the days went by, Adam gained weight, learned to drink from a bottle, and was able to come home. There was only one catch, however; he was to be sent home for the first year with a heart and apenea monitor; we were also to be trained on CPR. Well, they couldn't locate any monitors to send home with us, so, we had to sign our little boy out of the hospital each day and bring him back by 9:00pm until they found a monitor that we could keep at home. I call my little Adam, my Jesus, because we signed him out on Christmas Eve Day, and shortly after we returned him, they called saying they had found monitors that could stay at our home. We could come back and get Adam and bring him home for good; he was our best Christmas present ever! He got to come home with us on Christmas Eve!

Adam won his first battle in life only to endure a much bigger fight later in his young life. This fight is against Duchenne Muscular Dystrophy.

After we learned of Adam's diagnosis of DMD back in 1990, while stationed at Myrtle Beach AFB with his biological dad, Douglas MacDonald, we called everyone back home and told them the news. We all cried! When I was younger I used to collect money for Jerry's Kids and now I had one of Jerry's Kids. Because I had some prior knowledge of MD, I played a big part in Adam's diagnosis. I went to his pediatrician on base and told him what blood test to run, and he listened to me and told me that he didn't know much about neurological diseases. He did tell me that a new doctor had just been stationed at the base that did have some knowledge of neuromuscular diseases. He called the doctor who came to the office and took Adam over to a set of stairs. He had him walk up the stairs because he wanted to see how he managed the stairs. He also had him sit on the floor and get back up again. Adam used his arms to pull himself up the stairs using the railing one step at a time and he used his hands to crawl up his legs to go from a sitting to a standing position. This is called the Gower's Maneuver (which I knew about from watching the telethons over the years). Within the hour we had the results of the blood work and the diagnosis was Duchenne. We were then scheduled to have a muscle biopsy to confirm the blood work results. We were told that boys with DMD often don't live past the age of 16.He may never graduate High School and he would stop walking by the age of 12. Your dreams for your child as a parent get shattered when you hear these words.

Growing up as a child of a military member I didn't know my grandparents or other relatives very well and wanted to bring Adam closer to home so, he would get to know his grandparents, uncles, aunts and cousins. His dad cross trained in the Air Force from Aircraft Maintenance to Recruiter, and we were able to move to Brewer, Maine, which was only a 2 ½ hour drive from family. Within 2 years of moving back to Maine, Adam's dad left us. He stayed in Adam's life for a while, but slowly but surely has vanished almost completely from his life. Adam and I relocated to Presque Isle where family is on both sides. I completed the CNA (Certified Nursing Assistant) course, and have worked many hours at two jobs to support us. Adam enjoyed so many activities, and I kept him busy as I knew someday he may not be able to do things like snowmobiling, sledding, boating, Cub Scouting, fishing, hunting, camping, kayaking, and driving his all-terrain go-cart. He had to give up cable TV in order for me to afford the payments on the go-cart! He often went cruising with his friends along Main Street and he worked at the school farm for 3 seasons. Adam cleaned his own room and he loved helping me do dishes and fold the laundry. Besides being mother and son, we are the best of buddies. We did so much together and because I am now his full-time caregiver, we do everything together now. Adam walked until he was 14 years old. He had a Harrington Rod placed in his back at age 16 to correct Neuromuscular Scoliosis (most DMD boys have to have this surgery after they are confined to a wheelchair). It helps to straighten their back and keeps the rib cage from putting pressure against the lungs and other organs. Adam graduated from high school in June, 2004. He was the first male student to go across the stage and he received a standing ovation; everyone was standing, cheering, and clapping.

Another thing we did together was to jump right into fundraising, which we have been doing ever since Adam was diagnosed. Adam represented MDA as a State Poster Child in South Carolina and subsequently as a Goodwill Ambassador. We attended many MDA events, and also organized our own fundraisers. We also began to volunteer every Labor Day Weekend to answer phones and do live interviews on the local MDA Telethon. When we moved back to Maine, Adam once again represented MDA as a State Poster Child and has been a Goodwill Ambassador ever since. Last year we celebrated our 20th Anniversary of volunteering at the MDA Telethon. Adam has been featured in newspapers since he was a baby; it started while in England. The Children's Miracle Network donated funds for the hospital to purchase new incubators and Adam was the first baby in the ward to be placed in one of the new ones. The headline was *Little American baby boy first to use a new incubator.* He has been in the news media every year ever since for one thing or another, but mostly for MDA events, and recently for his attempt to raise $2,600.00 for Parent Project Muscular Dystrophy for his 26th birthday.

Awareness and Fundraising are so important in the fight against DMD. I am still saddened to say that Duchenne isn't well known like we families would like it to be. However, the world is slowly learning one person at a time about how devastating this disease is for a boy, and though rare, even girls can have DMD. We recently learned after my son went through an appendectomy, just how little is actually known about Duchenne. Our medical professionals often won't listen to us regarding our sons' care even though we are pretty much the experts up against someone who has never heard of DMD. Because of improper use of oxygen and pain medicines, Adam went into two episodes of respiratory failure and we came close to losing him. This year we were blessed to have surprised Adam with a 26th birthday party. Adam also continued his fight to raise funds for much needed research. He raised $3,646.00 for Parent Project Muscular Dystrophy, He once again exceeded his goal to raise a total of $2,600.00 for PPMD ($100 for each year he has lived with Duchenne). This is the 3rd year that Adam has raised money for DMD research for his birthday. When he turned 24 he went through Causes on Facebook to raise $2,400 for CureDuchenne, but he fell short and only raised $300.00. He wanted to give up after becoming discouraged that the public doesn't take Duchenne as seriously as they do cancer. But, we talked and we decided to try it again when he turned 25. This time we added a Birthday Party Fundraiser which was held at The Crow's Nest (a new restaurant that was just opening here in town). He also used Causes through Facebook and had some local publicity. Adam raised almost $10,000.00 that year for CureDuchenne. This year was the 3rd Annual Adam MacDonald Birthday Wish Fundraiser and he selected PPMD. Sadly, the fundraiser we organized didn't get much support from the community this year, but Adam did exceed his goal of $2600 by raising $3,646.00 for PPMD. Adam is happiest when he knows he is making a difference in his own life and the lives of others who are also battling the same disease he is!

The time is now for the world to take notice of DMD. It is time that Duchenne becomes a household term, and it is time for the medical world, especially pulmonary specialists, to learn about Duchenne in their college studies. My motto is that when you hear the word Duchenne or the words Duchenne Muscular Dystrophy for the first time, that you take time to research it and then do something about it!

*Cheryl Markey*

# Pete, 26 Years Old
# and Joe, Deceased

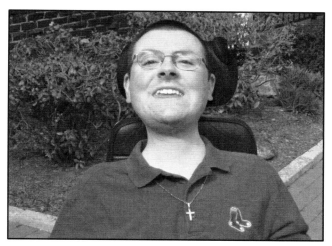

My husband Tim and I met in college fell in love and got married, and two years into our marriage, began a family. We were so excited to welcome Pete into our lives in 1985. Two years later Joe arrived. Life was good. We enjoyed family time so much. Each day was a gift. What a blessing our sons were to us.

When Pete was three we enrolled him in a cooperative preschool program. Pete was so excited to be with other children his age. This gave me time to do some things with Joe. As the year progressed the teacher expressed her concern to us in regards to Pete's gross and fine motor development She thought he should repeat the three year old program. We happened to mention this fact about Pete to the family doctor at an appointment for Joe. We also shared how Pete used his hands to push up on his legs to get into a standing position. We thought this was cute. We never read developmental books so we had no idea that this might not be typical. The family doctor just said, "Let me do a blood test on Pete to look and see if there is any problem with his muscles."

On Monday morning, four days after Pete's blood was drawn, the doctor's office called and wanted to see both Tim and I that afternoon. We knew that something must not be good for the doctor to want to see both of us. We arrived at this appointment and I blurted out all kinds of questions. Once I was done the doctor, in no uncertain terms, said, "Pete has Duchenne Muscular Dystrophy (DMD). This is a fatal disease and there is no cure for it." He explained a bit to us and then left the room to get the telephone number of a Muscular Dystrophy Clinic doctor in Boston, MA. We were in shock. When the doctor came back in the room he shared his concern for our other son as well. Joe was not walking and he was 18 months old. Joe's blood was tested and 3 days later he was diagnosed with DMD too.

Back in 1989 there was no internet. My husband went to the library to read about DMD the next morning. As Tim shared when he came back home, "it was like he was reading about Pete". He saw pictures and at three and a half years old Pete exhibited some of the same postures Tim was seeing in the books. Tim's heart ached like it never had before. Our dreams for our family and our sons were shattered. We would need to dream differently!

This was way beyond something we ever imagined for our lives. We had to put all our trust in God. We knew that there was no way we could do this on our own. As we learned more about DMD, we realized that we would need to move into an accessible home, buy a wheelchair van to accommodate our two sons' power wheelchairs, and go through a range of so many mixed emotions. As a Dad and Mom we wanted our children to be treated just like anyone else. They are people. We made a decision to make their lives as rich and as full as possible. We have had so many wonderful memories of all the activities and events that we all participated in. Some of the highlights have been hot air balloon rides, helicopter rides to visit special people and even small Cessna plane rides.

Through Pete and Joe's lives we have been able to enjoy and be thankful for so many little things. Their perseverance and determination taught us so much. They are our heroes.

Time seemed to be going by way too fast. Elementary school flew by, middle school days disappeared quickly, manual wheelchairs came, leg surgery arrived, power wheelchairs arrived, and scoliosis surgery was done and before we knew it high school was upon us.

High school was such an exciting period in Pete and Joe's lives but also a very tough road. On the one hand you tried to enjoy each day but on the other hand it forced you to think about the future and what would our sons do after high school. Pete excelled academically but struggled socially. Joe, even though he was younger, was beginning to have some significant challenges. Joe was getting so tired that he could only attend school part time in 10th grade and was not strong enough to go to school for 11$^{th}$ and 12$^{th}$ grade. Joe needed lots of sleep. His cardiac and respiratory status was very weak and eating orally was presenting some safety concerns. At this point Pete and Joe were both using bi-pap breathing machines at night along with the use of the cough assist machine at times during the day. Joe had a feeding tube inserted at the age of 16.

Joe had a serious respiratory virus in the fall of 2003 and was in the hospital for one week. In 2004 Joe had a cardiac event in the local emergency room and said to us, "I think I am going to die." Joe was airlifted to a larger hospital where he spent a week in the ICU unit. His heart was very weak. We tried numerous medications to help Joe. After one week the doctors said there was not much more they could do. They said "take Joe home and love him." At the time we thought we only had days or weeks left to have Joe alive. Well Joe was able to live a little over 3 years longer.

During Joe's last three years of his life he taught us so much. He was sad to leave his family and friends but never afraid to die. He enjoyed each day like it was his last. What an example of how we should all live our lives! He always asked about how everyone else was doing even though his health status was declining. This was a challenging time for Pete. Pete was older but it was like he was seeing his future through Joe's decline.

We enrolled Joe in hospice which helped our family so much. The team would guide us through some pretty tough emotional and medical struggles for Joe. As time went on we were able to keep Joe comfortable as he began to sleep more and more.

In the fall of 2007 Joe woke up one day and told me he thought he was going to die. He had all the signs of death and I was home alone. We always prayed that when the time was imminent we would know and we would all be together. Tim and Pete were able to return back home within an hour. We had powerful and unbelievable conversations with Joe and Joe shared his three wishes with us. We held each other's hands and prayed over Joe. Two hours later Joe was feeling better. It was amazing the rebound Joe had. This day was such a blessing even though it was one of the toughest days of our lives. Joe always said he wanted to live until he was 20. Well he turned 20 a few weeks later and in November, 2007 he went to his new home in Heaven. As we said good bye to Joe, we thanked God for his short but wonderful life. We miss him so. Even though it has been 4 years now our hearts still hold a special place and always will for Joe and his life.

Pete is 26 now and doing pretty well. He has joined Toastmasters (a public speaking organization) and enjoys this very much. Recently he was awarded the Toastmaster of the Year for the local club. Speaking in public has become so much easier for Pete. Pete continues to inspire so many people through the great young man that he is. Pete also writes poetry. One of Joe's wishes was for Pete to write a poem about him when he died and better yet a book of poems. Pete is up to 20 poems which have been a huge help in his grief journey. Pete has been able to share all his feelings and emotions through poetry.

We feel so blessed to have Pete and Joe in our lives. They have taught us so much and we are forever thankful. We have met many families that live with DMD. We continue to learn so much from those who have been down the DMD road ahead of us.

*Joan Lafferty*

## Duchenne Warriors

Ian Griffiths, Ricky Tsang, Scott Sands, Rebekah Davies, Carl Tilson, Ben Safford, Sam Safford, Anthony DeVergillo

> "Believe life is worth living, and your belief will help create that fact."
> ~William James

# Ben, 15 Years Old

## Life Lessons

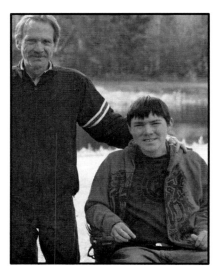

I'm Ben Safford and I have Duchenne Muscular Dystrophy. Although DMD forces me to depend on other people for almost everything, it is teaching me valuable life lessons. For instance, I have learned that a person's value does not depend on his physical strength or abilities, but on his spirit, character and heart. My greatest struggles are not physical ones, they are spiritual ones; like learning patience, forgiveness, and self-control. Without Duchenne, these life lessons would be harder to learn. Although I never would have chosen to have DMD, I know that it is an easier burden to carry than many other diseases people have. As a believer in Jesus Christ, I have learned to depend on Him and not to dwell on the fact that I have a fatal disease which cannot be cured. I look forward to having a home in heaven one day where I will have full use of my body.

*Ben Safford*

# Sam, 13 Years Old

## The "Real" Cure for Muscular Dystrophy

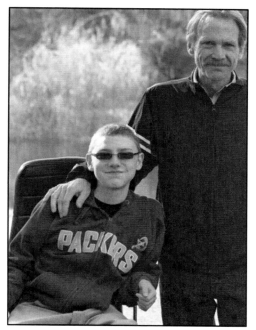

Hi, I'm Sam and I have Duchenne Muscular Dystrophy and there's no cure on the earth for it right now. I hope they find a cure on this earth, but I'd rather have other people get cured instead of me because the real cure is in heaven and I'm going there when I die because I'm a born again Christian and believe in Jesus. Here is a song by Jeremy Camp that talks about heaven. He wrote it after he lost his wife to cancer after only 5 months of marriage. Here it is:

**There Will Be A Day**

I try to hold on to this world with everything I have
But I feel the weight of what it brings, and the hurt that tries to grab
The many trials that seem to never end, His Word declares this truth
That we will enter in this rest with wonders anew

(Chorus)
But I hold on to this hope and the promise that He brings
That there will be a place with no more suffering
There will be a day with no more tears
No more pain, and no more fears

There will be a day when the burdens of this place
Will be no more, we'll see Jesus face to face
But until that day, we'll hold on to you always

I know the journey seems so long
You feel you're walking on your own
But there has never been a step
Where you've walked out all alone

Troubled soul don't lose your heart
Cause joy and peace He brings
And the beauty that's in store
Outweighs the hurt of life's sting

(Chorus)

I can't wait until that day where the very one
I've lived for always will wipe away the sorrow that I've faced
To touch the scars that rescued me from a life of shame and misery
O, this is why, this is why I sing

(Chorus)

There will be a day he will wipe away the tears
He will wipe away the tears
He will wipe away the tears
There will be a day

# Anthony, 18 Years Old

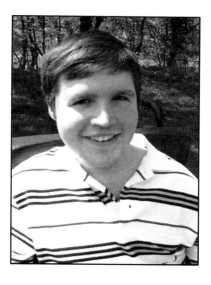

### Do Me a Favor

Do you think the sun won't shine?
Do you think life does not matter?
Well all that has to change,
Now it's time to rearrange,
Make your life really shine,
I found a way for everything to be fine,
Just do me a favor and smile.

Do me a favor and smile,
Be happy for more than a little while,
Let me see that gleam in your eye,
To let this feeling never die,
That look upon your face,
Is really all it takes,
To change the world.

With all the bad in this world,
It's time for happiness to be unfurled,
It does not matter who you are,
You can still shine brighter than a star,
Black or white,
Straight or gay,
A smile will surely change the way,
You look at every single day.

Some of you may think,
That life will always stink,
That you have to throw your dreams away,
That happiness can never really stay,
But just think back to the time,
When a smile was not a crime,
You were only 8 years old,
And life to you was diamond and gold.

Do me a favor and smile,
Be happy for more than a little while,
Let me see that gleam in your eye,
To let this feeling never die,
That look upon your face,
Is really all it takes,
To change the world.
I've seen it for myself,
How a smile can change a life,
Even if it's full of strife,
I have a disability,
Where everything is harder for me,
But then I figured out,
That happiness was the perfect way,

To a perfect life every single day,
And I wanted to scream and shout,
Tell the world what optimism was about.

And you can do the same,
Cuz life's not about money or fame,
Not about strife or pain,
Or what in your life you can gain,
It's about that simple look,
Upon your face,
That makes the world a better place.

*~Anthony DeVergillo*

## Carl, 24 Years Old

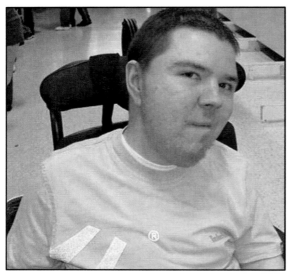

I have Duchenne Muscular Dystrophy at 24 years old. I was diagnosed at the young age of five. It all started with me falling over when my mother took me to see the general Doctor. He said I was just a late developer and that she was an over anxious mother.

It wasn't until I had trouble climbing the stairs when my parents took me to see the specialist doctor at the Children's hospital where they took a muscle biopsy which indicated I had the condition. Life in the family changed. My mother got depressed, especially after the consultant mentioned the word "terminal" suggesting we take photographs and videos for the memories as it doesn't look likely I'll make it past my twenties. Time went on and my parents came to grips with the harsh conditions. They pledged to give me the best life possible while showing me love and affection. I had a good childhood. I really enjoyed my trips to Disney World in Florida. There is something really special about that place that all children should experience. I started school and mainstreamed until I went into a wheelchair at 8 years old. Then I was taken to a special school which had all my needs in place. I felt very well supported at the special school. However, I've always thought my education would have been better in a mainstream school because I felt like I was held back in the learning department. I did however have excellent attendance and never hardly missed school unless of course I was feeling poorly or had a hospital appointment. I was a hard worker and passed all my exams. I wasn't great at math but I still passed, the subject I was most excellent at was English and computer technology.

In my last year of school I had an operation on my back as I had a slight curve of the spine so I had to have rods put into my back to correct the curve. It was a huge operation but I did get through it. The doctors were pleased with me. I am so glad I had it done, especially now.

When I finished school I went on to college to study computer technology and graphic design. I spent three years there. I would have been there longer if I didn't become so sick. I was rushed to hospital because I was finding it hard to breathe and my oxygen levels were dropping. Once there they got me on a bed and used a machine called a cough assist where a lump of phlegm came up that was lodged in my windpipe. The hospital found out the reason of my chest infection was because I was silently aspirating. This meant I had to have an operation to have a tube put into my stomach. I was in hospital for weeks. Once out I never went back to collage because I was too far behind. As time went on I found myself feeling depressed. During this period of depression was when I found Action Duchenne and became an active campaigner and spokesperson for Duchenne Muscular Dystrophy. I have never looked back since.

*Carl Tilson*

# Rebekah, 26 Years Old

## But You're a Girl....

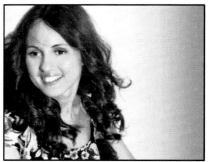

I guess you could say that most of my friends growing up were boys, most of whom had Duchenne. From a very young age, I knew only too well what this disease was and what it did. Little did I know that one day I would face the same fate.

I had always struggled to walk. I seemed weaker than other girls my age, but doctors told my mother that this was because I was born 11 weeks premature; despite the fact that I had all the classic symptoms of DMD.

Fast forward to my teen years. I could no longer eat without help and my mom was doing everything for me, from feeding and showering to scratching my nose! Doctors then told us they would run some tests. I went into the hospital for a week. They tested me for everything but DMD. After failing to discover what was wrong, they told us I had muscle weakness and sent me home. Without a diagnosis, my mom and I continued to live with DMD. I began to struggle with swallowing and breathing, and was rushed into the hospital to have a feeding tube placed. Still, the doctors where confused as to what could be wrong. I was sent home after spending 3 months in the hospital, but we were all still clueless. Even after two heart attacks and having to be put on a bipap vent, the doctors STILL did not test me for any type of MD!

One day in October of 2010, a blood test showed that I had high CPK levels, a trong indication of DMD. A few weeks later I was diagnosed with Duchenne. When I asked the doctor what took so long to discover my condition, he looked back at me confused and said, "Girls are not supposed to have this". We now know all too well that although Duchenne is rare in girls, it is not impossible. It does happen .I went home from the hospital that day and never once asked "why me?". Instead, I went out and partied with all my friends, to celebrate the fact that for 25 years I had lived with DMD and overcome every obstacle it had put in my way.

DMD has never stopped me from living life or for reaching for my dreams. Like any girl, I love shoes, shopping, fashion, and makeup. Am I ashamed to admit that to me image is everything? NO! I can tell you now that I'm more likely to be found worrying about what I am going to wear or where the coolest place is to be seen on a Saturday night, rather than the latest health risk DMD has brought to my continually weakening body. I mean, I might as well concentrate on the things that REALLY matter, Right?

I had always dreamed of becoming a model from a young age; however, I was never tall enough, nor could I stand up, so I guess you might think that I was doomed from the start. Well, think again. I used my disability to promote myself and a positive image of disability in general. I want other young people in the same situation as myself to look at me and think, "If she can do it, so can I". Nothing is imposable. Right now I am an ambassador for the Muscular Dystrophy Campaign UK. AND I LOVE IT. For me it's all about inspiring future DMD families to live life. If you have to live with this condition, it is better to work with it then against it.

I don't hate Duchenne. I have to live with it and smile. DMD does not define who I am; it is simply a small part of me. It has brought some amazing people into my life, most of whom I never would have known otherwise. Through this terrible disease I have found love and happiness, and above all, I have learned to make every second count. So for all you have brought me Duchenne muscular dystrophy, I THANK YOU.

*Rebekah Davies*

# Ian, 26 Years Old

## Excerpt from, DMD, Life, Art and Me

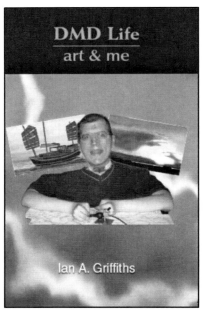

...being poked and prodded by the nurses, they asked for any medical history I had. Obviously I told them about suffering from "Duchenne Muscular Dystrophy". I also mentioned having mild asthma as well as telling them what had been going on over the past few days. Intravenous drips' were inserted into either arm with extreme difficulty. I have contractures at my elbow so straightening them is impossible as they are permanently bent at forty five degrees. All drips and blood taking are done on my forearms using very thin or "butterfly" needles. I had no idea what they were pumping into my bloodstream. My lungs were still hurting and I felt gravely ill, I was getting impatient because I wanted some relief from this ghastly sickness.

The hours dragged on slowly and painfully. I didn't know how they were going to improve my situation. My uncle Alan popped in to see how I was doing and to see if I was alright in the afternoon. At the time and while my family were watching a nurse called Helen brought in a long thin tube and explained that it was a suction catheter. She was planning on feeding it down my nose passed the back of my throat and in to my windpipe to try to clear the mucus from my lungs.

She attached the tube to the hospital suction and began feeding it down my nose. It was so painful; it felt like it was cutting all my air off. I could feel it snaking its way around the back of my throat and sliding through mucus membranes into my windpipe. The secretions were violently moving up and down my trachea and occasionally they would get stuck stubbornly, I just managed to move the blockage with a cough in time which increased the burning pain panging in my chest. She started the suction but after a few attempts she wasn't getting anything up at all it was too thick, my eyes started watering profusely. My ineffective cough started up and it was extremely hard to control.

Helen then removed the catheter to check on my progress. Two or three minutes later I turn to look at my uncle when out of nowhere another cough erupted. I felt a huge plug of mucus move in my trachea I tried to cough it out but it got firmly stuck. I tried desperately to breathe my lungs burst into pain as they ached for some life giving air. I tried harder and harder to breathe and the pain intensified beyond anything I knew. My heart pounded so loudly in my ears. I was drowning in a pool of my own fluid secretions. I knew something bad was going happen. Suddenly my eyes rolled back and everything went black at the same time my body slumped dangerously back. Was this the end of me, I thought I would surely die. I fell unconscious and to this day don't remember what happened next...

*Ian Griffiths*

# *Ricky, 30 Years Old*

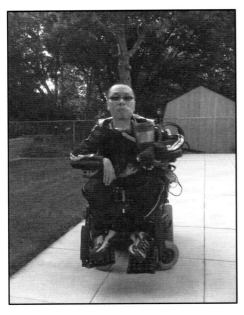

Dear Duchenne Moms,

There isn't a day that goes by when thoughts of you don't enter my mind. I write lyrics and tunes in literary melodies, but no words could describe the gratitude I have for you, your unconditional cares and affection. It moves me with heartache every time I think of your lifelong sacrifices, but in you is where my sanctuary lies, knowing that I'm loved, always.

Between the hardships and despair, the smiles and laughter still linger. They continue seeping through, like the radiance of sunlight; its warmth from within. In a walk that was never mine, you've taken my hand and challenges with it, making them ours without hesitation.

Through your enduring spirit of strength and courage, I've learned that sometimes, we have to stop crying and live. Despite physical limitations, you refuse to let me feel sorry for myself and have the luxury of self-pity. Instead, you encourage me with expectations that include neither condescension nor partiality. With only dignity, grace, and a tremendous amount of gentleness and patience, you've given me a newfound respect for women that will stay with me forever.

Although I'm one to shatter dreams when you lay eyes upon my frail abode, I understand your fear of the future to come. This is reality, and as I fall apart to the notions of breaking your heart, I'll stand tall, even while the world crumbles in my sight, for you've taught me well. I live for myself and am not afraid, because hope remains with me.

And I'm sorry I can't relieve your burdens, for not being able to prove my love. I'm sorry for a lot of things. I hope you know that words for me often speak louder than actions. I might never be able to reach out and hug you, but if I could, I would... do anything for you. You've given your life to me and all of mine is yours.

But this isn't about apologies. There's nothing to be ashamed of when we're in this journey together. No obstacle has existed in vain. It isn't about thank yous either when you've asked none from me in return. I only hope that I've become the man you envisioned me to be, both in my heart and soul.

Dear Duchenne Moms, I nevertheless thank you for loving me throughout the years of my life. It's nearly impossible for another to love me, but yours is my inspiration to understand that if our roles were reversed, I'd love and take care of her, just as you did me. Perhaps in this, you may remember that hope rests upon my foundation in you, and because of you, I know what love really means.

Remember me, for who I am, for you're my mother, and I'm your son. I always will be.

With hope,
Ricky

# Scott, 42 Years Old

## Taking A Bow From The End Stage - by Scott Sands

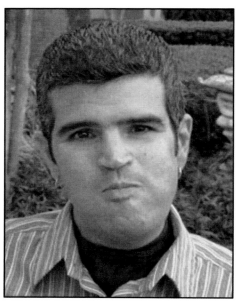

Duchenne muscular dystrophy experts and clinicians have isolated me into a category that I absolutely detest – *End Stage*. I never particularly cared much for that term, especially when it is associated with yours truly! Why? Well, *End Stage* tells me that I'm essentially *old*. *End Stage* implies that I'm a lot closer to the finish than I would like to be, like some aging baseball player winding down his career as a tired, broken, overweight, pinch hitter. *End Stage* indicates that I'm in grave condition and might as well start knocking on death's door because it won't be long. *End Stage* says just that – nearing the *end*. I am close to the end of life, the end of love, and the end of pleasure and pain and possibilities. The end.

If you go with the textbook definition, then yeah, I am in the *End Stage* of Duchenne muscular dystrophy. Yes, my heart is bad. Yes, my lungs are screwed. Naturally, at this point in the disease, I have progressed about as far as I can go just short of, say, maggot food. I am under constant watch by nurses and never left alone. If a tree farts in the woods, can anybody hear it? Yeah, my nurses can - they hear everything! They are trained to notice my every little nuance, every ventilator alarm, every change in color, every sneeze, every *ouch*, every swallow, and everything else. Plus, I have a team of physicians monitoring my condition and ready to intervene if I go awry. And I could easily go awry on a moment's notice, like the time I suddenly went into complete heart block! Indeed, you will find my picture in the dictionary under *tenuous*.

Heck, doctors were giving me the *End Stage* spiel when I was twenty-three! I didn't buy it then, and I certainly don't buy it now! Duchenne is way too unpredictable. Some die at ten. My brother did not get past fifteen. Others reach thirty. I am forty-five and still crushing odds. I am not in this part-time; I am in it for the long haul, baby!

Regardless, though, the inevitable question of mortality will ultimately stare you square in the eye.

My very first confrontation with a Duchenne death was the passing of my brother, Joseph, when I was eight years old. But a child sees things in simplistic form. I knew that Joseph had a disease and couldn't walk. I knew I had the same disease and *could* walk, albeit not as easily as the other kids. I knew that Joseph was in the hospital and I knew when he died there. I attended his wake and funeral and I realized that I would never see him again. However, that was a brush with *Joseph's* mortality.

My initial confrontation with my *own* mortality came when I was 23, at a rock concert of all places. It was on a chilly October night at the old Shea Stadium in New York. My brother, Nick, ushered me through an endless maze of blue police-barricades outside leading to the gate during a persistent drizzle. We met up with my best friend, Jimmy, in the disabled seating area out on the first tier, which would be the right field porch at Mets baseball games. On this night, the Rolling Stones hit town, and were ready to blow away the packed house! And we were prepared to rock all night long with Mick and the boys!

As my brother darted into the long line at the concession stand to get a beer, Jimmy and I sat impatiently waiting for Living Colour – who were set to open for the Stones on this leg of the Steel Wheels tour – to take the enormous stage in centerfield. Just then, a big, burly, wheelchair-pushing, paraplegic dude in a tank top rolled over and began to engage us in some typical pre-show banter. Like many male paras, he was built like Hercules up top and a stick figure from the waist down, and had an ego as large as his pectorals.

Anyhow, the dude chatted briefly with Jimmy before turning his attention to me.

Para: "Hey, this should be a great show, huh?"

Me: "Yup."

Para: "I'm John." (He extended his hand, but then quickly tapped my shoulder when he noticed that all I could muster physically was an eyebrows' wiggle of acknowledgment.)

Me: "Scott."

Para: "Pleased to meet you, *Steve*. So, what's your disability?"

Me: "Uh, Duchenne muscular dystrophy."

Para: "For real? Wow! I didn't know you guys lived *this* long."

Wake up call. Reality check. Slap…in…the…face!

John's single remark served as a brutal reminder that my days were indeed numbered and that I actually *had* a limited life expectancy. Prior to that altercation, my life at the time was all about sports, music, college and co-eds and beer. Impending death wasn't even a thought. But the dude managed to put a bug in my ear about a Duchenne reality that I had been unconsciously ignoring. His obvious alcohol-induced interrogation was downright nauseating! I swear I would have smacked the guy if I had enough strength to raise my right arm! What was even more annoying was his medical ignorance. But really, who could blame the dude? Like most people, all he knew about muscular dystrophy came from Jerry Lewis on the MDA Telethon. He was aware that he had muscle and we did not, and that statistics said we typically died young. Little did I know then that I would dodge all the Duchenne bullets and still be here over twenty years later. If John saw me today, still kicking, he would probably suffer a massive coronary! You see, muscle isn't what makes you tough; gumption does, and I definitely have plenty of *that* to go around!

I never looked at DMD in *stages*. As far as I'm concerned, there are only two *stages* for each of us – birth and death. Anything in between is just called living. Life is an elevator; it has ups and downs. Have you ever seen a stage? It's typically flat. Actors perform on it. Musicians play on it. Dancers twirl on it. Orators speak on it. Politicians lie on it. The Stones *still* rock on it, but I don't hear anyone telling Mick Jagger that he is in the *End Stage* of anything, and the guy is ancient!

Indeed, I am one of the older DMD patients on record. But what the expert clinicians and scientists don't know is that I spit nails, I don't take any crap, and I am a survivor of the fittest. And I eat DMD for breakfast! Count me out, will they? Number my days, will they? Rest in peace? Me? Ha, no way!

So here I sit, stuck in a seemingly perpetual *End Stage*, and I am taking a bow!

*Scott Sands*

# Rest in Peace Our Duchenne Heroes

"Some Angels have wings and some have wheels!"
*Unknown*

# *Dylan Smith, 12/14/96 – 10/17/11*

### *Living on the Edge*

(A story written just a couple weeks prior to Dylan's passing by his mother Melanie Mackie. Dylan was only 14 years old.)

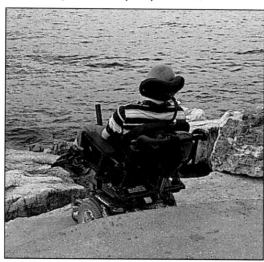

It was a shock to hear the doctor tell me I was pregnant. I never planned on being a MOM at this point in my life. I was scared, but at the same time I was excited. Nine months passed quickly and the time came to deliver my son into the world. The labor was intense, and to this day I wonder if he knew what was to come. He did not want to come into this world. I tried; I pushed for hours. Eventually the doctor pulled him out, cut the cord around his neck, and hoped he would start breathing. I brought him home and totally fell in love. He learned all the normal things a toddler should: how to eat, talk, play, walk, and even run. He was a perfect baby; He was a happy baby; and he was a very cute baby.

Dylan's third birthday came and something didn't seem right. He was pale, constantly wanting to drink water, and continually peeing thru his diaper. I took him to the doctor and after some convincing; he agreed to do a blood test for Diabetes. I looked it up and read about it while waiting for the results. I was hoping it was not a positive blood test. My family, Dylan, and I went out for dinner the evening the doctor received the results. Dylan's blood sugar was very high, 55. Even though it was very high, he was still alert and seemed ok. At the hospital, the nurse gave him a shot of insulin. It brought his sugar down way too fast and he started vomiting. After a week in hospital, trying to absorb a ton of information, we went home. This was January of 2000, a month after he turned 3. I have to say I really don't know how I did it, but I managed to pick this up right away and keep his sugar levels under control. He started eating 6 times a day and getting needles every day. This part took him quite some time to get used to as did the finger pokes to check his sugar. Juvenile diabetes doesn't run in my family, so it was a big shock to us, but I dealt with it because what else could I do?

Less than 3 years later, Dylan was diagnosed with Duchenne Muscular Dystrophy (DMD). He originally got very sick with gastroenteritis (a very bad flu) and was admitted to the hospital. The ER doctor decided to do several blood tests, one of which came back showing extremely high liver enzymes. At this point the doctor thought something was wrong with his liver. We ended up at *The Hospital for Sick Children in Toronto, Ontario.* Dylan had to endure a liver biopsy. This was scary for me as I didn't like him being put under for this procedure. Thankfully it was done very quickly. This procedure turned out to be completely unnecessary because there was nothing wrong with his liver. Dylan's diabetes doctor decided to ask them to do a blood test to test the muscle. Sure enough, they found his CPK levels to be very high. On September 3, 2002, one of the worst days of my life, Dylan was diagnosed with DMD .

From this day on everything changed in my life and also in Dylan's as well. After learning how to walk, he was now about to learn that he would lose that ability. It turns out that when a child has a life- threatening illness, they can have a wish granted to them. Dylan wanted to go to Disneyworld and meet Mickey Mouse. Make a Wish took care of everything. We got to ride in a limo, fly on a plane, stay in Florida at an amazing place called Give Kids the World, go to all the parks AND have some extra spending money. It was the best; Dylan had a great adventure. Dylan's decline in muscle strength was a slow process. You would think this was a good thing, but it wasn't. He started using a walker and then went to a manual wheelchair, and finally having lost his own independence, he got an electric wheelchair. He was actually very happy to get the electric chair after several years of struggling. The power chair was his prize. Dylan will be 15 on December 14, 2011. The time seems to have just flown by. I wanted to share with you all of the vehicles Dylan has been in because he is proud of all of them. He loves anything with wheels. His ultimate favorite is the city bus),but he has also enjoying riding on a train, plane, boat, 18 wheeler, smart car, tow truck, fire truck , ambulance, taxi, limo, jeep, pickup truck, cars, accessible race car, moving truck, ferry, school bus, steam train, snowmobile, go-kart, pontoon, police car, coach bus, zoo-mobile, hay ride wagon, riding lawn mower trailer, golf-kart , ATV, mono-rail, subway, two accessible vans and a convertible!

At this time Dylan's heart is being damaged by Duchenne. It is pumping and working so hard to keep him going. This disease is evil and I sure hope a cure can be found so that other kids will not have to go through this. Dylan doesn't know he is dying, and I will remain positive and fight the fight as long as possible for him. He will laugh right up until that time because he is so innocent and his personality makes him shine. Life with DMD is very exhausting and emotional for me but I have to stay strong for my son. He needs me right now and I will not leave his side. I will continue to pray for a cure, but I'm afraid it will be too late for my Dylan.

*Melanie Mackie*

# Matthew James Frye-Vidovich, 6/7/94 – 7/11/11

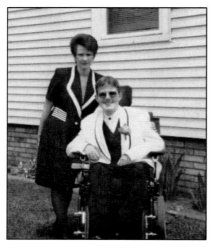

Matt was a strong man even though he could not move a muscle. Matt was a gentle man when he could have been very bitter. -All that was Matt. Because he chose to go through the narrow gate; he chose Jesus.

There is a peace that can only come through acceptance.

Acceptance is not giving up; it is not throwing in the towel. It is finding peace right where you are at and pressing on ward. I am sharing this because my hearts cry is that we do not linger long in despair, but that we dance in the rain, we find joy in today…tomorrow will come and we can deal with it then. Live like there is no tomorrow, stand tall and let the Creator carry the burden. Joy is in your laugh, smile and shout. Do not let the worries of tomorrow cloud your thoughts today. Be blessed everyone. Find joy…right where you are today.

*Doreen Vidovich*

I was Matthews's mother, caregiver and friend. We laughed and cried together. I was blessed to be his mother, and blessed to be able to take this journey with Matt right till the end, when he left to be with Jesus, he is in his care now.

# Joe Lafferty, 9/22/1987 - 11/18/2007

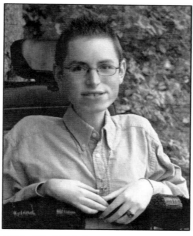

### A POEM FOR MY BROTHER

You were quite a bro
And you let it show
You were always super courageous
With a smile that was contagious

All of you Joe loved
And he flew like a dove
He now soars like an eagle
Not like an ordinary sea gull

You we will miss
And we'll blow you a kiss
You were so brave
And not death's slave
You were quite a joy
Ever since you were a little boy
From a special friend you loved a hug

With your Red Sox blanket you were snug

You loved dogs and cats
And looked cool in hats
You liked the Pats
And rooted for those guys with the Red Sox caps

Now when I see a rainbow
I'll think of God's promise to you
You now have eternal life
And no more strife

You are the champ
And we loved going to Joni Camp
You're now in heaven
And it's you we're craving

You were so good
And you sure enjoyed food
You were never in a bad mood

You loved meeting babies
Your new life is sweeter than candies

You lived life with such grace
And now you've won the race
Oh how we miss you so
You were quite a bro

*Pete Lafferty*

# *John Nagle, 1980-2007*

## *Medical Negligence: A Duchenne Horror Story*

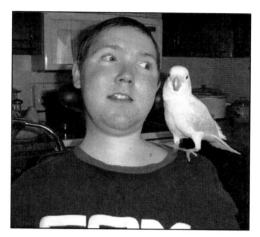

I'll never forget the moment I laid eyes on that adorable little boy. I fell in love with him when he reached out for us with his tiny arms. When Social Services informed us that he had a form of Muscular Dystrophy, which turned out to be Duchenne, we had to make a choice that would seem difficult to most. However to us, there was no other choice than to bring him home to call our own.

John had a special place in everyone's heart. He was a joy to be around, and wise beyond the not so many years of his life. He loved his family very much.

He was a genius in the creative arts; incredibly knowledgeable in the infinite aspects of the entertainment industry, always providing information on the latest films, music, and technology associated with it. We looked to him for expert opinions and he never ceased to amaze us with his insights into a world he found at the tip of his finger. He was a poet who diligently worked to produce the ultimate screenplay, and his enthusiasm for life was never tempered by what many saw as a devastating disability.

But fate told a different story on the early morning of April 28, 2007. John spent most of the night before chatting with friends on the internet and at five o'clock; he asked to be put to bed. He was only able to rest for a short while as he needed to use the commode.

After putting him to bed once more, I immediately had to transfer him back to the commode and the same thing happened. Within an hour, he wanted to try again as he complained of being constipated. He rested some more following his efforts, but with much discomfort. At two in the afternoon, he started complaining about pain in his lower-right abdomen. Thinking it could have been gas, I tried rubbing the area since it had occasionally helped in the past, but the pain worsened and by five o'clock, he wanted to be hospitalized.

I couldn't get him up into his wheelchair because every time I tried, he felt as if he was going to pass out. I called for an ambulance so they could keep him flat, and he was transported to the local hospital. When he arrived at the emergency room, he was given an intravenous line and they tried to get his blood pressure up with little success. They inserted a tube into his neck area in another attempt, but with great difficulty, trying a number of times. They also did a CT of his lower abdomen but found no obstructions. He was catheterized but had little output. The doctor told us the outcome looked grim and that he wanted to transfer him to the Intensive Care Unit.

During that time, I had been in contact with a doctor we had seen once at Children's Hospital in Washington, D.C. He recommended that John be transported to another D.C. hospital. He thought it could have been a gastro problem and the gastro doctors at their hospital were at a conference.

Although we specifically told them not to use oxygen, they put John on it anyway. He was taken via helicopter but I wasn't allowed to accompany him on the flight, so we drove there and met him at the emergency room. He was terribly uncomfortable being fluid filled and heavy, but had no urine output, yet they continued giving him fluids to bring his blood pressure up. He was taken to the ICU at nine o'clock in the morning but still had the same problems. Despite their lack of records, many scratched their heads trying to determine how they might proceed.

Fluid filled and with almost no blood pressure, they intubated him at eleven o'clock. I was told to leave the room and got ushered outside to the waiting room while they did the procedure. I tried gaining access to John but was not allowed in the room.

At about two in the afternoon, I saw John for a few moments. I believe the intubation wasn't done correctly because he didn't think he was going to make it. He went into cardiac arrest, and although they tried to revive him, they were not successful.

My son, John, died that day because of medical negligence. Why didn't they call the doctor who was the Muscular Dystrophy Clinic Director, or at the very least try to contact his primary care physician from Children's? Those doctors and medical professionals, whom I trusted, were making uninformed decisions, knowing little about Muscular Dystrophy or about John. They gave him morphine for the intubation (standard procedure, but not for people with Duchenne), and tried to intubated him without air. Even while John insisted that he wanted me to be there, they refused to honor his request.

He never wanted me to leave his side, but I was denied the right to direct them, knowing what they shouldn't do but did. They just wouldn't listen. I could have spent more time with my son, but they wouldn't let me see him for more than three hours straight. By that time, it was too late.

While I struggle with the anger and sadness that still consumes my heart, I'll continue living with hope and an upbeat spirit. John's last wish was for me to continue the MDA Yard Fair, an event held annually at the Farmer's Market in Charlotte Hall, Maryland, that has raised more than $100,000 for the Muscular Dystrophy Association.

"Do it as long as you can," my son told me.

This story isn't meant to bring people down, but to make them aware. I hope this never happens again, to anyone. I hope you'll help spread the word. And you might think it was silly of me to adopt John, considering the future complications, but if I had the chance, I'd do it all over again. I never saw him as a boy with Muscular Dystrophy.

John was born on October 4, 1980, adopted when he was ten months old on August 11, 1981, and he died on April 29, 2007. John Vernon Nagle was my son and my inspiration. He always will be.

John contributed twenty years of his life to promoting the worthy cause of the Muscular Dystrophy Association in an effort to find a cure. The screenplay of his life shall continue in hope, for others.

*Janet Nagle*

# Duchenne Story Contributors For Ages 0-10 Years Old

**Katherine Palmer:** My husband and I just recently discovered that our son, Andrew, has Duchenne MD. I am a stay-at-home mom living at Ft Campbell, KY, where my husband is stationed with the Army. There is no history of muscle disease in my family so Andrew's diagnosis was a shock to us. Neither my husband nor I knew anything about Duchenne (or any form of muscular dystrophy) before our son's neurologist mentioned it as a possible underlying cause for Andrew's weakness. Now, knowing what I do about DMD, I feel that I have a responsibility to spread awareness and to do what I can to help find treatments for it. Right now, while my son is too young to take part in clinical trials, that means raising funds for MDA and educating whomever I can about muscle disease. I also believe that God has a reason for bringing DMD into my family and that, as a Christian, I need to help others affected by this disorder turn to Him. I hope that my story in this book can bring a sense of comfort to someone else out there with a Duchenne child and remind them that they are not alone. We can do all things through Christ who strengthens us! You can follow along with me and my family's journey with Duchenne at www.HomemadeTaterTot.blogspot.com.

**Jeanette Wood:** Daniel's mom. I am the wife to my best friend, Joseph Wood. Together we have 11 children; six that were born from us physically, and five that were born from our hearts through adoption. We love to share our lives with others in hopes that we encourage them and offer them hope as so many have done for us. You can visit me online at: www.amomentwithmom.com or on facebook at: www.facebook.com/Momentswithmom

**Elaine Cabe:** I am Aidan's mother. When I found out about Aidan's diagnosis, the only thing that really helped was to hear other people's stories, what they feel and how they dealt with life. I started blogging and then I met Misty. Our blog is www.thecabejourney.blogspot.com.

**Jon and Kira Mullaly:** Have been together since high school and have always wanted a large family. They have 4 children (one with Duchenne) and live in Southern New Hampshire. Jon is a Paramedic and Kira is a Sr. Software Quality Assurance Engineer. Jon is also a testicular cancer survivor. We hope that one day Duchenne will be a household name and we believe advocacy, knowledge and education is key to a cure for Duchenne. http://www.our-mix.blogspot.com/

**Donna Anderton:** I am a fortunate woman to be happily married to Matthew for the last eight, wonderful years and am looking forward to many more. Together we have three beautiful children, Mitchell, age five; Cooper, age four; and daughter Reese, age 15 months. I am a primary teacher who is now a full time stay-at-home mum. I now have to use these skills I have acquired throughout my career to guide my kids and family through these uncharted *Duchenne* waters of our future! As a proud Australian, I hope to try to advocate for the *global awareness* for Duchenne Muscular Dystrophy. I have a blog at www.the-andertons@blogspot.com or directly email me at: mdmcra@bigpond.com

**Kristen McGourty:** I am the proud mother of 4 1/2 year old Liam and 2 1/2 year old Abigail. As a Pediatric Nurse Practitioner in a large practice near Boston, she was familiar with Duchenne Muscular Dystrophy from a clinical aspect, but never dreamed she would be grappling with it is as a mother. Liam was diagnosed in 2009 with DMD and since that point in time; Kristen has been a tireless advocate and fundraiser for DMD. She strives every day to give Liam and Abby a full and happy life, to keep her family together, to raise awareness, and find a cure for this dreadful disease. In what little spare time she has,Kristen likes to participate in triathlons and road races, and help new moms learn to breastfeed in her work as a lactation consultant at a Boston area hospital. Despite the challenges she faces, Kristen always has a smile on her face and the willingness to help others.

**Seavey Castelli:** Wife of Jim Castelli, and mother of two beautiful children; my twenty year old daughter, Crystal and my 4 year old son, Chase. I am submitting my story to help get awareness of Duchenne out to as many people as possible. I would like awareness to reach medical professionals as well. There seems to be a total lack of Duchenne knowledge in the realm of general pediatricians as well. I feel that if they are more educated in Duchenne and MD in general, we may get help to a lot of these boys sooner. My son was diagnosed by accident and only because I was pushing doctors to figure out what they were missing. I want a cure found in THIS generation.

**Stacy Daniels:** My husband, Jimmy, and I met during our freshman year in college and were married in 1991, the same year we graduated from Florida State University. We moved to Georgia where Jimmy received his law degree and where we are currently raising our seven beautiful children, four daughters and three sons. Two of our cherished blessings (our two oldest sons) were diagnosed with Duchenne Muscular Dystrophy in 2010. Our middle son has a dual diagnosis of DMD and autism. In addition to keeping up our wonderful household, I am involved with other families with special needs children in our community and with several organizations such as MDA, CureDuchenne, PPMD and Autism Speaks.

For more information as well as regular updates on our boys, please visit our blog: http://danielsclan.wordpress.com or find The Daniels Clan on Facebook: http://facebook.com/danielsclan and show your support by clicking the "like" button. Above all, we ask for your prayers! Thank you, and may God richly reward you for taking action to END DUCHENNE!

# *Duchenne Story Contributors For Ages 11-15 Years Old*

**Ben Polhemus:** Along with Jill, Kyle, Ellyse, and Ayden; I live in Valparaiso Indiana. I am a pastor at Liberty Bible Church and Jill is a dental hygienist. As a family we enjoy movies, eating, cooking, outdoor adventures, and storage unit auctions. We are submitting this story to share how Duchenne has done its best to ruin our lives, but it hasn't, and we have become stronger as a family because of it. www.fathersohope.blogspot.com

**Kelly Frangella:** I am a single mom of 4, 2 boys and 2 girls. My baby Carlie has Duchenne Muscular Dystrophy. I love gardening, camping, floating and my kids. I want the world to know that girls do get Duchenne, and I want the world to know about my Carlie. Awareness is the key to Funding, and Knowledge of this disease by non-affected people. I tell everybody that will listen. Carlies Crusaders@webs.com - research donations, Carlies Crusadors.webs.com - personal donations, Carlies Crusadors on Facebook under Health and Wellness

**Laura Villeneuve:** If you want the basics, here they are. My name is Laura Ville-neuve and I am thirteen years old. I believe that sending in a story to SOSD2 is important because I will be in a book with lots of other people who may or may not be going through the same process I am. I also wanted to do this because I always tell my brother's 'story'; and I wanted people to hear my side of his story. You can contact me at: karavee@comcast.net

**Kerry Gutierrez:** I am Seth's mom. Seth was diagnosed almost four years ago. It has taken me awhile to accept having DMD in our lives. For Seth, the signs of DMD have been minimal for the first years since diagnosis. I feel that has kept me almost in a denial phase. Getting to be involved with parents, research, or advocacy wasn't something I was able to do because that would make DMD a reality. Recently, Seth has entered the transition phase. This has been my wake up call. I have decided to do as much as I can to speak out to others and make them aware of DMD and what it is doing to our sons. The effects of DMD are taking ahold of Seth rapidly and I now see the limited time I have to try to save my son. I think putting Seth's story in SOS&D2 will be a way for me to reach out to family, relatives, and friends. This will help them to better understand DMD and what it is doing to Seth and other children. I hope as they gain knowledge, they can pass it along and we can find new hope in a cure for this generation of DMD children.

**Gretchen Egner:** I'm a high school English teacher, originally from Rockford, IL, but have lived in Mukwonago, WI, for the last 20 years. I have been married to Brian Egner since 1991, and we have two sons, Alex, 14, and Nick, 12. Nick has Duchenne. Since 2005, I've been running with PPMD's Run for our Sons team. An admitted couch potato until adulthood, I've logged 2 Full Marathons and 6 Half Marathons raising money and awareness to fight Duchenne. I'm a firm believer in seeing what's in the glass rather than lamenting about what's missing or what's not "fair". Life is good.

**Robert Alm:** I am the father of two wonderful sons who have Duchenne, Jackson and Hayden. I was informed of this venture by my ex-fiancé, who is the best mother that my boys could ever expect to have and is also the best advocate that I have ever seen for the cause of aiding and curing kids with DMD. I am telling my story for a number of reasons. First and probably least important, is the fact that not many dads write about it, although from personal experience, I can assure you that they care just as much. Men just don't talk about it, something to do with our gender I imagine. Secondly, I believe that this issue is one that is not just pressing but has a need to be aired. I think that it must be! Also, I think that too many times, all that is said about muscular dystrophy is all of the hardships and turmoil on both the children and their parents, when there are so many wonderful things learned by both parties by going through this process. I have never seen so much giving, caring, bonding, and loving in my entire life. This disease changes not only the children it affects, but those close to them as well, and for the most part, in a good way. Yes, your life changes significantly when faced with this challenge. There are sadness, anger, frustration, guilt, and even unhappiness, but this is all outweighed by the rewards that you receive.

**Lori Safford:** Mother of Ben, Sam and Lydia. After receiving my MA from Simmons College in Communications Management and working in the field of marketing communications for 17 years, my husband, Mike, and I made the decision for me to stay home full-time after our children were born. It is the best job I've ever had! I love volunteering at our small Christian school, attending school events and chaperoning field trips. I enjoy volunteering at Make-A-Wish (www.newhampshire.wish.org) events and for Joni and Friends (www.joniandfriends.org), an organization that meets the needs of families with disabilities. I co-lead a Moms Morning Out group for moms of kids of all ages with disabilities of all kinds. During the final editing of this book, I lost my beloved husband and my children lost the most loving Dad they could have ever had. We miss you terribly Mike, but I promise to honor you by caring for our three precious ones with every ounce of love, strength and grace God gives me. My life is certainly not what I ever would have planned, but it is a good life. I can be reached at lorisafford@comcast.net.

**Ben Safford:** Is a vibrant 15-year old who lives life to the fullest. He enjoys reading, politics, academics, singing, video games, and bossing his younger siblings around. He lives with his brother, Sam, his sister, Lydia, and his parents in Southern NH.

**Sam Safford:** Sam is a joyful 14-year old living with Duchenne in Southern NH. He loves to watch the Green Bay Packers, hang out with friends, play video games and drums. He hopes to get his band, Solid Serpent, off the ground one day soon. Sam is often caught in the middle between his older brother Ben, and his younger sister, Lydia.

**Star Bobatoon:** Her greatest accomplishment is being the proud parent of 'two of the most beautiful children in the history of children." Her youngest is her daughter Xanthia and her eldest is her son Hurricane. Hurricane has Duchenne Muscular Dystrophy and is the inspiration for her book *I Hate Muscular Dystrophy*. Star is an accomplished attorney, dynamic trainer and award-winning speaker whose high-energy and engaging style makes a lasting impact on her audiences and clients. Star's background in employment litigation and diversity counseling allows her to connect with diverse audiences, further enhancing her effectiveness as a speaker, trainer and executive coach. Star has also trained with and shared the stage both nationally and internationally with world-renowned motivational icon Les Brown.

Star is especially committed to organizations that support parents with special kids. She is a volunteer, speaker and workshop leader for informal support groups and national organizations including Parent Project Muscular Dystrophy (PPMD), Muscular Dystrophy Association (MDA) and the Make-A-Wish Foundation. For more information about Star Bobatoon visit www.IHateMD.com or email Star@IHateMD.com.

# Duchenne Story Contributors
## For Ages 16-42 Years Old

**Brenda Morea:** I am Joey's mom. I live in Searcy, Arkansas, with my husband of 26 years, Jeff, and with our son, Joey, and our youngest daughter, Amanda. My oldest daughter, Amber, and her husband, Evan, have blessed me with my first grandchild, Kaiden. My middle daughter, Joanne, is stretching her wings and is on her own for her first time. I am excited about being in this book, as I want to help everyone to see the value of our kids, to see what a gift they truly are. I also love to advocate for Duchenne, and I am planning to have some websites and blogs soon. I want to help educate about this disease and offer support for others dealing with it. If you would like to contact me, my email is brendamorea@hotmail.com.

**Margie Saliba:** I am Eddie's mom. I am a registered nurse, working for Partners Healthcare at Home, married 20 years to Edso, who is retired from the Massachusetts Laborers Union Local 223. We have two children; Eddie, who is 19, is a second year college student at Quincy College; Maggie is 18 and a freshman at the University of New Hampshire. As a family we have advocated tirelessly for 15 years, raising awareness and funds for Duchene Muscular Dystrophy, but we haven't done it alone. Throughout it all, countless numbers of people have supported our cause and, in the process, have become better educated about the challenges and obstacles that families of children with neuromuscular diseases face every day. Most importantly, we have shown our children that anyone and everyone has the power to make a difference. Through the incredibly hard work, support and love of organizations like the Jett Foundation, the Muscular Dystrophy Association, the Parent Project, Cadillac CureDuchenne and the National Football League, we can continue to offer our son the best quality of life we can, treatments at some of the top hospitals in the world and hope—hope for a cure for this horrible disease.

**Misty VanderWeele:** I am Luke and Jenna's mom and Glen's wife. I have authored 3 Duchenne books. *In Your Face Duchenne Muscular Dystrophy All Pain All Glory! Saving Our Sons One Story at a Time,* and now this very book *Saving Our Sons and Daughter II.* I am on a mission to create an army of Duchenne Parents, siblings, family and friends in what I call the Duchenne Movement. You can also find me in the book, *Celebrating 365 Days of Gratitude.* It is time the world knows what Duchenne is. That is why I am committed to global Duchenne recognition. You can learn more about me at http://MistyVanderWeele.com. Be sure to check out my all new e-magazine, *THRIVE! —In the face of Duchenne Muscular Dystrophy* while you are there.

**Cheryl Markey:** I was remarried on May 10, 2008 and my son Adam has DMD, diagnosed back in 1990 while we were living at Myrtle Beach A.F.B SC with his biological dad. We moved back to Maine to bring Adam closer to family as I grew up in the military and didn't really know my relatives and wanted Adam to know what a gram/gramp, cousin, aunt/uncle was. His dad left us in 1993whenwe were living in Brewer Maine, so, Adam and I relocated here to Presque Isle where his grandparents live and some of his uncle/aunts and cousins.

**Joan Lafferty:** I am honored to write this story as I think about all I have learned through the lives of my precious sons and just want to share so people can under-stand that there is joy in the journey. I live in Nashua, NH, with my husband, Tim and my son, Pete. Our other son, Joe, died four years ago at the age of 20. I have been married for 29 years and am thankful to be able to be the primary care giver for my sons.
Each day I am thankful for the gift of life and the memories that our family has been able to share. No matter how challenging my days can be I am grateful for everything and treasure all that I have learned through Pete and Joe's lives. What true blessings and precious sons!

**Anthony DeVergillo:** I am an Optimist. A few months ago I started a blog called The Optimist's Guide to Life at http://www.anthonysabilities.com/blog/ that has over 12,000 first time visitors in only 10 months and has reached all over the world, from California to Australia. I love working on my computer, helping others, and striving to make the world a better place for everyone. I have a never give up attitude and believe that having Duchenne Muscular Dystrophy is actually a good thing for me since it taught me life lessons and brought me on an Optimistic journey that has made me who I am today. The following poem mostly describes my Optimistic journey and why I spread Optimism in the first place.

**Carl Tilson:** Fighting adversity is the game, Action is my name. I'm an active campaigner and spokesperson for the condition Duchenne Muscular Dystrophy. If I'm going down, I'm going down fighting!

**Rebekah Davies:** I am 26 year old female with DMD, yep you guessed it I'm one of a kind, or as I like to call it limited edition as you probably know this rotten disease is mainly present in boys. Duchenne Muscular Dystrophy has taken me on quite a journey with major bumps in the road along the way. Despite all the twists and turns in my life I am living for right now and embracing all that DMD throws at me, be it good or bad, I'm too busy living to let it stop me from achieving my dreams. I'm a full time applied Psychology student and model as well as an ambassador for the Muscular Dystrophy Campaign Uk. Friends and family call me a professional princess like it's a bad thing I love being a girl shopping, shoes and makeup, never mind my ventilator I couldn't live without lip-gloss!! However I believe, "Beauty is only skin deep. I think what's really important is finding a balance of mind, body and spirit. "live every night as if it's your first and every day as your last" "There are no regrets in life, just lessons" "I have nothing to rub out no regrets" A very special man once said to me "Duchenne muscular dystrophy may destroy my body, but it will never destroy my spirit! " and baby I couldn't agree more!

**Ian Griffiths:** aka, "thebigG22005" Digital artist. Check out my art at www.ArtWanted.com/thebigG22005

**Ricky Tsang:** I'm a new author from Ontario, Canada. I was diagnosed as a six-year-old boy in 1988, but yet refuse to be defined by Duchenne Muscular Dystrophy. In my book, *RIDICULOUS: The Mindful Nonsense of Ricky's Brain*, I want to show people that anything is possible, despite physical limitations. It's important to emphasize our abilities and I thrive on making people feel good about themselves, for in that there's always hope. And I hope you remember me, for my words and who I am.

# Duchenne Story
## Rest-In-Peace Contributors

**Melanie Mackey:** I am from a small town of Collingwood in Ontario Canada. I wanted to write a story about my son Dylan's life to of course tell what DMD boys go thru (some allot worse) AND of course raise awareness about this rotten disease Duchenne. Things may have been different if he didn't also have the Diabetes but was not the case. Dylan passed away October 17th 2011. It was peaceful and in our home because that's what Dylan had wanted. He did not know he was going to die and he fought so hard till on that morning he did not wake up. He was in a coma. The two diseases just didn't work well together at all his heart function decreased quickly. He is my strength and my angel son from heaven and was the best kid you will ever meet. He had touched so many lives in his 14 years. So many. His funeral was full of love and sadness of course and the church was full of so many people that cared so deeply. You are all forever in my heart. We all miss Dylan so much and I know I will see him again one day. WE NEED A CURE FOR THIS DISEASE DUCHENNE MUSCULAR DYSTROPHY!

**Doreen Vidovich:** I was Matthew's mother, caregiver and friend. We laughed and cried together. I was blessed to be his mother, and blessed to be able to take this journey with Matt right till the end, when he left to be with Jesus, he is in His care now.

**Pete Lafferty:** Pete is a 26-year old young man with Duchenne. He lives with his family in Nashua, NH, and enjoys writing poetry, speaking, and serving as emcee at Joni and Friends New England Family Retreats.

**Janet Nagle:** I live in Southern Maryland and have lived here my entire life. My husband and I have been married for thirty-nine years. We both wanted children and adoption was our option after learning that biological children were not possible for us. Our first child, John Vernon Nagle, we adopted after ten years of marriage. John was nine months old and had been diagnosed with Duchenne Muscular Dystrophy at birth. My story is about the medical debacle he faced during the last day of his twenty-six years of life. We also adopted a daughter about ten years after John. She was nine years old. She has been a blessing as a daughter to us but also as a wonderful sister and friend to John. Our family has supported the efforts of the Muscular Dystrophy Association for the last twenty-five years with an event to raise money for medical research. It is our hope that research will bring an end to this disease. Our memorial site for John Vernon Nagle can be found at www.somdmda.org. It includes some information about our event and pictures and poetry written by John, our precious son.

# Honored Duchenne Heroes of Past

Michael Bryan Rivera born September 21, 1980-February 20, 2007

Travis Edward Gordon was born January 27, 1991-November 25, 2011

Ronald (Ronnie) Michael Shatto born November 19, 1985-June 6, 2010

Jarle Jacobsen born October 5, 1981-September 16, 2011

# Epilogue

Through these heart-felt, often times heart wrenching, personal Duchenne stories, the world needs to understand that a cure MUST be found for Duchenne. Duchenne is a progressive muscle disorder that causes loss of body function, independence and eventually loss of life. To date, there is no known cure and can happen in any family. We need your help to change that. —WE CAN'T STOP NOW! Our sons and daughters need us! To learn more about the Duchenne Movement or to support our cause, please visit.

*MistyVanderWeele.com*

## Saving Our Sons & Daughters II - Duchenne Movement Affiliate Program.

A portion of the proceeds of *Saving Our Sons & Daughters II* will go to the co-authors who chose to become a Duchenne Movement affiliate. Such affiliates selling books will earn a commission based on books they sell. Such commissions can go towards expenses insurance won't cover, pay bills, give to their favorite Duchenne charity or to use toward something special for their Duchenne children. Herby any commissions earned by the affiliate/co-author will be spent at their digression and are liable for any taxes due on such earned commissions. For more details about the Duchenne Movement Affiliate Program contact Misty VanderWeele at misty@mistyvanderweele.com.

# Duchenne Books Published
## by Misty VanderWeele

*In Your Face Duchenne*

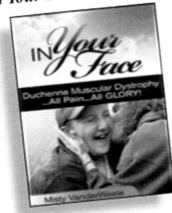

*Saving Our Sons*

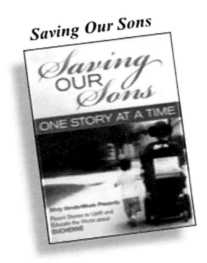

**"Beacon of light to others who face the same challenges" Patti B.**

*In Your Face Duchenne….!* NEWLY REVISED AND UPDATED….Duchenne Muscular Dystrophy wasn't going to stop this mom from living the best life possible. Misty shares openly the roller- coaster of Duchenne in this heart touching, surprisingly laugh provoking book In Your Face Duchenne Muscular Dystrophy All Pain All Glory! A book she has written in celebration and preserving her son's essence while he still graces her life with his presence. A gift to present to him for his mile stone of high school graduation and more importantly staring death "in the face" with triumph and success.

*Saving Our Sons One Story At a Time,* First Duchenne-Parent Collaboration book of its kind. Where parents come together to share their personal stories as a way to shout out the SOS call to the WORLD, that *A CURE MUST BE FOUND!*

**Quality Paperbacks Available**
**Order Online MistyVanderWeel.com**

# *I Hate Muscular Dystrophy,*

## *Loving a child with a life altering disease.*

### ~Star Bobatoon, Esq

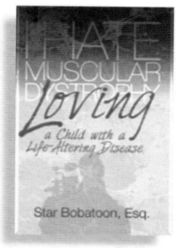

"Life is not about waiting for the storm to pass but about
learning to dance in the rain." ~Anonymous

"Why me?"

Was the question Star Bobatoon asked when her 5-yr old son was diagnosed
with Duchenne Muscular Dystrophy.

This book is an authentic story that speaks of the strength and resolve of a
mother who believes that life is to be lived and celebrated, despite any real or
perceived limitations.

www.IHateMD.com
It is also available on Kindle and
Nook.

# Ridiculous

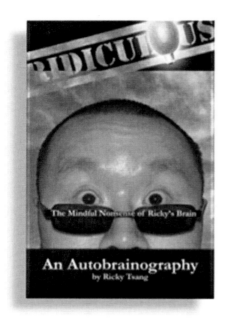

## Ridiculously Romantic

## Ridiculously Hilarious

## Ridiculous
*Mindful Nonsense of Ricky's Brain*

Without focusing on physical limitations, it's a book about the things we're capable of doing; the freedom within who we are. Packaged in a chaotic mix of romance and comedy at its finest and told with brutal honesty and heartfelt emotion, Ricky Tsang's uncompromising style of redefining the infinite facets of life promises to keep readers on the edge of their seats.

Hilarious, original, and refreshing… it's absolutely and unequivocally RIDICULOUS. Available now on Amazon.com and in e-book format, get your copy TODAY.

**For more information, please visit:
http://www.rickytsang.ca/book/ridiculous/**

# *DMD Life art & me*

## 25 years of my life living with Duchenne Muscular dystrophy,,,

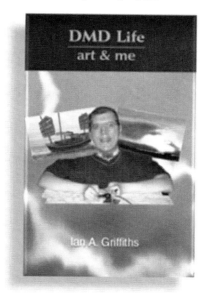

**Even though Duchenne takes so much away from those who suffer with it, there are things it can't take!**

"IAN has Duchenne Muscular Dystrophy the doctor tells my parents, a severe, fatal muscle-wasting disease that will lead to an early death. This is a chronicle of the first twenty five years of my life living with DMD read through as my ability to walk disappears, as my breathing deteriorates, as my heart fails and as I become increasingly paralyzed. Despite all the ventilators and mini tracheotomies I've still got my positivity and determination to see me through. I'm fighting back by campaigning and lobbying all the while helping a charity try to rid the world of Duchenne forever."

**Quality Paperback**
**Order Online DuchenneMen.net16.net**

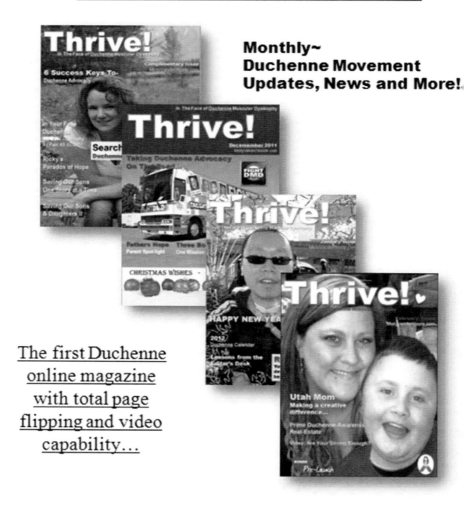